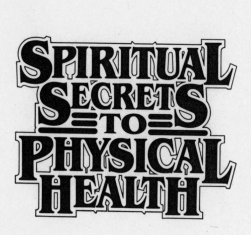

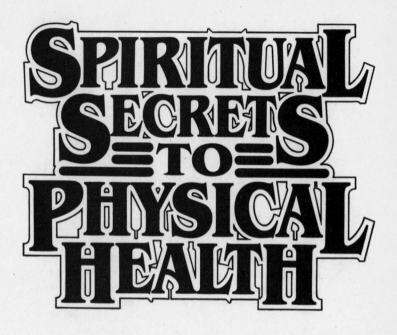

SPIRITUAL SECRETS TO PHYSICAL HEALTH

Paul Johnson M.D.
with Larry Richards

WORD BOOKS
PUBLISHER
WACO, TEXAS

A DIVISION OF
WORD, INCORPORATED

Library of Congress Cataloging-in-Publication Data

Johnson, Paul, 1915–
  Spiritual secrets to physical health.

  1. Health—Religious aspect—Christianity.
2. Spiritual life.   3. Spiritual healing.   4. Mind
and body.   I. Richards, Larry, 1931–
II. Title.
BT732.J64   1987   261.5'6   86-32551
ISBN 0-8499-0554-0

7898 BKC 987654321
Printed in the United States of America

Contents

Introduction

I've known Paul Johnson for more than a decade now and have come to value him as a brother, as a friend, and as a sensitive healer. We worked together earlier on *Death and the Caring Community,* a book about ministry to the terminally ill patient. Now I'm excited to have a part helping with a book much closer to Dr. Paul's heart—staying well.

As a Christian and as a physician, Paul Johnson views illness and death as enemies. For more than forty years he has been committed to helping his patients get well and stay well.

In this book Dr. Johnson shares what he has learned in his four decades of battling illness. He gives you what he has given his own patients: medical and spiritual secrets of recovery and vital good health. If you're struggling with illness or simply want to live a healthy, vigorous life, what Dr. Johnson has to share can enrich—and lengthen!—your life.

Paul Johnson's years of practice in Seattle have won him more than the appreciation of his patients; they have also earned him the respect of the medical community. Today, although retired from private practice, Dr. Johnson is a medical consultant to the State of Washington Department of Social and Health Services. And Dr. Johnson represents all of King County's 3,300 doctors on a weekly radio program.

Dr. Johnson's credentials are reassuring. What he shares with us in this book is not some fad or medical quackery. Doctor Johnson represents the very best in medical practice, enriched by a sensitivity to spiritual realities which grows out of his own faith and his experience as a healer.

That's what makes this book so significant. This is not

7

just a book of theory. It's not a book about fads. This is a book that has grown and matured as Dr. Johnson's own healing skills have matured, and as he has become aware of the healing powers that God has planted in every individual—powers that faith can and will enhance.

In this book you'll meet many of Dr. Paul's patients. You'll see the principles he teaches illustrated in their histories. And you'll find a number of medical nuggets as well—fascinating bits of information usually available only to those on the "inside" of the medical community. But most important, you'll learn how to apply Dr. Johnson's spiritual secrets of health and vitality to your own situation!

These well-established spiritual secrets will give you a basis for renewed hope of recovery from even the most serious of illnesses. And they will provide a pattern for daily choices that will lead you, like thousands of others, to vibrant good health.

LARRY RICHARDS

SPIRITUAL SECRETS TO PHYSICAL HEALTH

1

Being Well

I believe we were meant to be healthy.

That's one reason why it was always such a pleasure for me when Ron, a third-year medical student at an eastern university, dropped in at my office.

Ron's a handsome young man—outgoing, popular, athletic. And Ron was making all the right moves. He was making good grades, yet took time to play and relax. He had lots of friends and seemed genuinely considerate of those around him. Every time I saw Ron, I couldn't help smiling—thinking that here was a young person who was "well" in the fullest sense of the word.

One day Ron met a cute girl on campus, and they hit it off from the start. They began spending a lot of time together—playing tennis, swimming, going to movies. They even started planning for a shared future.

It seemed like an ideal match.

But there was something Ron didn't know. Jane was seeing someone else at the same time. She honestly liked both men, but she had to make a choice. It was hard for her, but finally she decided—against Ron.

Jane told him as gently as she could. But the rejection hit Ron like the proverbial ton of bricks.

Somehow Ron—healthy, hardworking, successful—had never experienced this side of life. And he couldn't handle it. Ron became depressed. He couldn't study and lost interest in tennis. He couldn't seem to care about anybody or anything, and he felt constantly tired and listless.

After about two months, Ron began to have some tingling on the right side of his face. A few days later his face was painfully inflamed, and the rash was punctuated with little blisters.

Just one look told me. Ron had come down with shingles, a condition that can be very serious when it occurs near the eye. In fact, to protect that eye, Ron had to drop out of medical school and be hospitalized.

What had happened to that bursting good health? What had happened to vital, vigorously youthful Ron?

I've seen it many times in my years in medicine. Ron's basic problem was a broken spirit. That broken spirit and his inner turmoil over Jane's rejection literally depressed his immune system to the point where he was vulnerable to the shingles virus.

Ron's physical illness was real. But I am positive that if he had been able to handle his breakup with Jane in a different way, he would not have become sick.

Body and Soul

It's ironic in a way. Today it's mostly the medical world—not the religious community—that's drawing attention to the relationship between body and soul. Multiple articles and studies demonstrate this basic reality:

Your body simply does not function well unless your soul and spirit are in a healthy, harmonious state.

The biblical vision of the human being as more than a material self is finding unusual and unexpected support. Many in medicine today share my conviction that we cannot treat the body without attempting to treat the mental and spiritual dimensions as well!

It's easy today to demonstrate the unquestionable link between physical health and the inner state. For instance, persons under unusual stress are much more prone to develop ulcers. When all your systems are functioning well and in balance, and when you're in a healthy emotional and spiritual state, a layer of mucus insulates your stomach from your digestive juices. (If you've ever wondered why those stomach acids that dissolve the medium-rare steak you ate for dinner don't eat out your stomach lining, now you know!) In the stressed individual, however, stomach acids are more concentrated and the normal mucous layer protecting the stomach lining actually disappears, resulting in ulceration.

Simply put, stress—and your response to that stress— can throw your body's systems out of balance. The interaction of the prostaglandins, endorphins, enzymes, hormones, and many other chemical systems that work together to keep you and me healthy and feeling well can be thrown out of balance.

When that happens, you're in for trouble! Back and neck aches, headaches, nausea, dry mouth and flushed face, knots in your stomach, cramps and diarrhea, dizziness, pounding pulse, rapid breathing, and even chest pain can come simply because your psychological and spiritual response to stress has upset your body's physical systems. Thousands of hormones, enzymes, and chemicals are out of balance—some systems flooding you with too many chemicals and others not functioning at all.

When that happens, you're a prime target for a serious and potentially disastrous illness.

The Answer Is Within ══════

It fascinates me as a doctor to realize that the body, soul, and spirit are so closely linked.

Why? Because if much of the illness I treat has roots in my patients' souls and spirits, then treatment of the soul and spirit holds tremendous promise for healing!

At one time, I assumed that if I performed necessary surgery and prescribed antibiotics and other medicines, I'd reached the limit of what I could do for my patients. But gradually I realized that if I took the time to know my patients, took the time to discover what they were experiencing within, I could do more! Gradually I discovered that the secret of recovery for most of my patients lies within their minds and hearts, not in their bodies. Gradually I learned some of the spiritual secrets that lead to recovery and make for a lifetime of vigorous good health.

Actually, I suppose you could say I learned from my patients.

Take Mrs. Hull, for instance. She was seventy years old when she came to me with a pain in her stomach. Examination showed that she had a very large malignant tumor of the stomach.

By the time I saw her, the cancer had spread so far that there was no way to operate and still have a live patient. Still, I did a palliative removal, cutting out much of the main mass in order to prevent bleeding and obstruction. Mrs. Hull did very well during her postoperative course and left the hospital without knowing the extent of her disease.

She was such a pleasant lady. It really hurt me to sit down with her family after the operation and tell them the whole story. And it really hurt to give them my prognosis—I was sure there was no chance for Mrs. Hull to recover.

I fully expected Mrs. Hull to show up at my office any

day with an extension of the tumor. But week after week, month after month, she didn't come. Finally I called her home. She was eating well and, she said, "feeling just fine."

After a year, I convinced Mrs. Hull that we should take x-rays of her stomach to see what was going on. To the amazement of everyone involved, *there was no evidence of any tumor!* Her stomach looked as if nothing had ever happened.

Much later I understood.

Mrs. Hull had a strong faith. Her entire family gave her love and support. There was never any doubt in her mind that she would get well, so her inner being or spirit was always secure.

I had just stood by and watched the power of a healthy spirit promote healing!

Mrs. Hull lived into her nineties. And when she finally died, her death had nothing to do with cancer.

Avis, a nurse I've known for at least twenty-five years, is another amazing example. She has always been outstanding in her profession as night supervisor of a large Seattle hospital. I became her physician, and I learned to respect her for her nursing expertise and her personal lifestyle. We had a very good doctor-patient relationship.

Before she retired, Avis volunteered for a five-year breast cancer prevention program, in which a group of women had regular breast examinations and also an annual mammogram. Avis was always faithful in her examinations and finished the program one August. The following December she came to me with a large mass in her left breast and an axilla filled with enlarged lymph nodes. She had cancer, and a very virulent type.

Avis was positive about the whole thing. It was then I learned that she is an earnest Christian with a deep trust in God. Never once during her course of treatment did I see her give in to despondency or doubt—a truly remarkable display of faith. Her treatment wasn't fun and games, but she came through like a champ.

It's been seven years now, and Avis is positive that she is cured. All the tests we have been able to do show that she is probably right.

Of all the cancer cases I've had, Avis should have done most poorly. She had an aggressive, rapidly growing tumor that had all the marks of being uncontainable. But today Avis is cancer free. And although she gives credit to conventional therapy, she is as sure as I am that without her faith she would not be here to tell her story.

It's fascinating. A strong, healthy young man is broken by disappointment and develops a serious illness. A pleasant seventy-year-old with inoperable cancer recovers and lives into her vigorous and happy nineties. And a nurse with one of the most virulent forms of cancer known undergoes her treatment with a quiet faith—and wins.

Yes, the answer is within.

A healthy spirit does promote physical healing. There truly are spiritual secrets to recovery and to living a healthy, vigorous life even into old age.

I've Been There ═══════════

I feel very strongly about the spiritual secrets I share with you in this book—not only because I've spent my life helping others recover from illness and stay well, but also because I've personally experienced many of the things I plan to tell you.

I was busy in my surgery practice in Seattle, totally involved in all the problems and rewards of dealing with people. It was past time for my own routine checkup, but I was busy. When I finally found the time, I learned I had cancer of the colon.

Needless to say, that news really hit me hard. I wasn't ready for it. I always thought it happened to the other person, not me. Suddenly my cozy world had been invaded by an enemy, and I was no longer in control.

It was nine o'clock in the morning when I got off the examining table and slowly dressed, trying to pull my thoughts together. One thing was sure. My previous plans were scrapped. All my priorities were changed. I would have to stop my practice and give full attention to myself. For years I had been ministering to others who were down. Now it was my turn.

That first day was a total loss. I was in shock. I knew that I was in for a long course of treatment, and that chances were I would never be able to return to practice. I knew the disease and what it might do. And I knew that I must have surgery immediately.

Later, after I'd said my good-byes to my family, I was carted to the operating room and transferred to the table. I recognized the surgery crew, and we exchanged some small talk. Then the needles went into my arm, and the anesthesiologist began counting as he started the Pentothal.

The next thing I remember I was falling in pitch blackness. I was in free fall, and somehow I knew there was no bottom. It was like falling into a black abyss. I felt alone and deserted, with nothing between me and total destruction. I had never felt so alone before. I was falling faster and faster, with no possibility of coming out of this one. I was absolutely terrified!

And then I seemed to hear a voice I recognized. It said, "Don't worry, Paul. No matter how far you fall, I'm here. I'll catch you." And I realized it was the voice of Jesus.

You can't imagine how much that relaxed me. I didn't care anymore how far I fell. All was well.

The next thing I remember, I was back in the recovery room. The first thing I told my wife, Genevieve, on returning to my room was my encounter in the free fall. I remember every detail to this day.

Just a hallucination? You be the judge. But I do know that the confidence I had in my surgeon and the experience I had in my free fall helped create a positive attitude. And I know that a positive attitude is one of those spiritual secrets that promotes recovery.

My surgeon showed me the pathology report. There was no doubt my tumor had spread, and some cancer had been left behind. With chemotherapy and radiation, however, I had a chance for recovery.

But by this time I was convinced I was going to win. I was helpless, but far from hopeless. And that is so important. Our immune system and our ability to recover is so dependent on our attitude. All the repair systems work at super efficiency when the gloom is lifted.

How many times had I seen it in my practice? Now I experienced it in my struggle with my own cancer. Along with my basic faith and confidence in God, I applied other spiritual secrets that I'll share with you in this book.

That was eight years ago. Today, as far as anyone can tell, the cancer is gone.

Actually, painful as it was, my illness proved a great gift to me. It not only confirmed many things I had come to believe about healing; it also gave me a fresh appreciation for life. My priorities now are based squarely on life's important issues, and I don't take wellness for granted. Life is beautiful and fresh, something to be enjoyed. My family and friends are very special to me. And my relationship with God is especially secure. What more could anyone ask?

But that's about my recovery. What about my illness? Why hadn't my immune system protected me in the first place? I don't know for sure, but I have a pretty strong idea of what happened.

Not long before my cancer was diagnosed, I had done surgery on a very close friend. It should have been routine. But twenty-four hours after surgery, he was running a high fever, and in forty-eight hours he was dead from the most virulent and aggressive infection I had ever witnessed. Massive antibiotics and life support systems had done nothing.

That incident so distressed me that it affected my entire life. I couldn't sleep, eat, or function. I was happiest working, but even there the memory of my friend's death constantly gnawed at me. I developed headaches, ringing in the ears, and nausea. I looked to God for comfort and release, but felt cut off from Him. My prayers went nowhere. In fact, I *couldn't* pray.

I went on vacation, but when I got away, the memory was still there with me. I just couldn't run away from my distress.

After a few months, I started to feel more stable. But one morning as I dressed for surgery, I noticed the skin of my abdomen and groin was broken out in giant hives—an indication that my immune system was seriously affected. I took medicines to control the hives and was able to carry on.

But inner distress takes its toll, one way or another. I'm convinced that my cancer had its origin in that incident and in the way I responded to it.

Mainline Medicine?

A few years ago I hosted a daily morning radio talk show. One day at 7:40 A.M., while I was on the air, the news director rushed in with a news flash that quoted the prestigious *New England Journal of Medicine*. It had just been discovered, the bulletin said, that carrots prevent cancer!

He asked me on the air, "What do you think about this, Dr. Paul?"

If I was sleepy before, that startled me to attention. The ball was in my court to make a statement to a lot of commuters on Seattle freeways and thousands more just waking up. No explanation was offered, just the head-line. What could I say? After a slight pause, I replied, "Well, pass the carrots." *ha!*

Later I read the journal article. It stated that caro-tene, a substance found in carrots and other foods, aids in cellular defense against cancer and is necessary for a healthy cell state. That was hardly a momentous bit of knowledge; we've known it for years. Carotene is con-verted into Vitamin A, which is vital for complete nutri-tion. Thus, carrots don't actually prevent cancer in and of themselves, but the Vitamin A produced by the caro-tene found in carrots does promote healthy cells, which could serve as a defense against cancer.

This is the kind of headline the media thrives on, and we the public are bombarded daily with truths, half-truths, and downright falsehoods. Today, medical items in the media have a number-one rating, outstripping even professional sports. No wonder we're flooded with medical spots, whole TV specials, and everything in be-tween! In our fast-paced and competitive society, the media will often "discover" something that's been around for years. They'll make a feature story out of it that gets national or even international attention—for a day, at least.

I don't want you to think that what I'm sharing with you is "new," or an amazing "discovery" that no one has ever realized before. And I don't want you to think that I advocate a "faith" approach to healing that rules out doctors and medicine.

The fact is that medical literature documents nearly everything I'll say to you in this book! And much of that literature and research comes from men and women who aren't particularly religious. Let me share just a few quotes with you.

Dr. Bernard Siegel, of the Yale School of Medicine, argues that "it's when people are attacked by feelings of loss and defeat that the body becomes ripe for disease." In an interview with *The Terrytown Letter* (No. 46, February 1985), Dr. Siegel says, "If everybody could learn peace of mind, by whatever means, we'd be so far ahead. People would see that they don't have to get heart attacks or cancer. Even high intensity Type A personalities would get things done and run businesses with less strain. I think this is the key issue: let people maintain their own identity. But teach them how to deal with *living.*"

The same issue quotes Dr. Herbert Benson, Associate Professor of Medicine at Harvard Medical School. Dr. Benson is Director of Behavioral Medicine and Head of the Hypertension Section at Beth Israel Hospital, one of Harvard's main teaching facilities. His 1975 bestseller, *The Relaxation Response,* has helped make meditation and prayer legitimate medical techniques. Partly because of his work, the National Institute of Health now recommends meditation techniques for blood pressure and stress problems. This is particularly important because the new field of psychoneuroimmunology shows that stress reduces the body's ability to fight disease, while an open trusting frame of mind enhances it.

Dr. Benson, who shows in his newest book, *Beyond the Relaxation Response* (Berkley Pub., 1985), that religious faith makes meditation more effective, doesn't recommend ignoring the miracles of modern medicine. Rather, he says, "the crucial point is to integrate medical techniques with our own powers of healing, to combine what medicine can do for us and what we can do for ourselves."

Dr. William Wilson of Duke University's Department of Psychiatry goes even further. In a lecture given at Loma Linda University in 1984, he stated that he believes firmly in the supernatural and is convinced that a personal relationship with God is basic to a healthy inner spirit. Indeed, he feels that a growing relationship with God is central to healing and "can be applied and have therapeutic effect" on biological problems as well as psychiatric problems.

Jane K. and John P. Dixon write with no religious biases. They say that "four crucial lifestyle determiners with demonstrated relationships to health have been identified."* These are *activity* (responding to an unpleasant situation by taking action to seek changes), *flexibility* (openness to new experiences), *integrity* (making choices that are in harmony with a person's sense of who he is and what his needs are), and *transcendence* (having the sense that life is oriented toward purposes greater than oneself, whether this involves God, human welfare, or some more limited cause).

All these researchers and articles are saying a very simple thing.

Health isn't just a matter of medicine.

Staying well is based on more than the hereditary advantages or disadvantages you were born with.

And getting well doesn't depend just on what a medical team does to you in the hospital.

In researching this book, I tied into the central medical computer in Bethesda, Maryland. There I found literally thousands of articles that say it again and again.

You are a whole person, not just a body. Your physical being is linked inseparably to the psychological and spiritual "you." Health is a matter of psychological and spiritual wholeness, not just a matter of how well your biological machinery operates.

That's why I wrote this book. I want to share with you what many in our medical establishment know—but all too many doctors ignore.

I want to give you the spiritual secrets—the principles leading to psychological and spiritual health—that can

---

*"An Evolutionary-based Model of Health and Viability," in *Advances in Nursing Science*, p. 1, April 1981.

make all the difference in your recovery even from the most serious illness and make all the difference in your experience of a vital and vigorous life.

I've taught these principles to my patients for many years. I've applied them to my own life. And I'm convinced they *do* make a difference.

An Amazing Machine

It's all too easy for us in medicine to forget that it takes a healthy spirit to promote healing. We so easily become caught up in the mechanics of the body.

Take your heart for instance. In your seventy or eighty years of life, your heart will beat some 2.5 to 3 *billion* times. It beats at the command of a specialized area of tissue located in the right atrium, called the sinus node. That node emits a positive electrical charge, which travels through both upper chambers of the heart. The impulse activates another area, called the atrioventricular node, which upgrades the signal and transmits it to the ventricles through special nerve filaments called the Bundle of His. The upgraded electrical charge is discharged into the muscles of the right and left chambers of your heart, causing them to contract and to pump the blood that nourishes every living cell in your body. All this is accomplished in a fraction of a second. Truly, as the Bible says, we are "fearfully and wonderfully made" (Ps. 139:14).

Modern technology has enabled us to study these electrical impulses. By applying wire leads to the chest, we're able to map the pattern of impulses on an electrocardiograph. We can diagnose heart abnormalities and monitor patients in intensive care units. The electrical charge and discharge is so constant and follows such a regular basic pattern that any abnormality can be discovered and problem areas can be pinpointed.

It's exciting for me to see the development of such medical tools. But what we've discovered while using this tool is fascinating, too.

Your heartbeat is actually initiated by nerve signals that originate in your midbrain, and your sinus node is controlled by chemicals known as catecholamines, which originate in the hypothalamus gland. These control your pulse and blood pressure automatically; you and I have no conscious control over the pumping of our blood.

Still, what we do has an impact on the heart and its electrical system. When we exercise, for example, the sinus node increases its rate of impulse discharge. Too much coffee will irritate the node. But an even more negative impact comes from smoking. Nicotine causes the node to discharge erratically, and the pulse becomes irregular, with extra or "premature" beats. Cigarettes are actually as disruptive to heart function as drugs such as amphetamines and barbituates. In fact, whatever drugs we take have an effect on the very center of our existence—the sinus node.

Our Choices Make a Difference

Medical truths such as these have driven home to me the fact that the choices we make, like our basic inner attitudes, have a definite impact on recovery from sickness and on staying well. I've seen this proved over and over in my practice.

John is a commercial painter. He'd been an alcoholic for many years when he became my patient, and I had seen him in his alcoholic state many, many times. Then, about twenty years ago, he came in drunk again.

It was one time too many. I was pressured and upset that day, and so I decided that was it. I told John I couldn't do anything for him and that I didn't want to see him again.

"But, Dr. Paul," he objected. "You're my doctor. And I need you."

I had no confidence in John at all, but I sat him down and pulled up a chair. "OK," I said, facing him. "Here's what you've got to do. You've got to ask Jesus into your life, to take your life over. That includes all your habits—especially alcohol."

"Please go over that with me one more time," he said.

Very carefully and slowly, I went over the gospel with him and talked about the power involved.

And John said, "I'll do it!"

He left then, and I fully expected he'd be back within several days, drunk as usual. But he didn't come back.

About a month later he dropped in—cold sober. He said he just wanted to let me know that he hadn't had a drink since I had seen him last. His parting shot was, "Why didn't you tell me about Jesus a long time ago? His medicine is a lot more effective than yours."

John's been dry now for over twenty years. During that time, he's not only joined a church and become an elder, but is very active in helping other alcoholics.

I learned a lot from John. In particular, I learned another category of spiritual secret.

You see, there's more to recovery and staying well than developing confidence and hope—more than learning how to build a positive attitude. You and I have to realize that the choices we make have a powerful impact on our physical health. The lifestyles we choose can enrich or impoverish us. And the lifestyles we choose can undoubtedly lengthen or shorten our lives!

When a doctor moves beyond fascination with the mechanics of the body and moves beyond reliance on the wonders of medical technology, he or she comes face to face with basic reality: *The real key to health and well-being is the kind of person who lives in a body, not the bundles of nerves and muscles, the chemicals and glands, which compose it.*

At the beginning of this chapter I wrote, "I believe we were meant to be healthy." I do. I believe that God gave you and me bodies that were equipped with the resources we need for a lifetime of vibrant good health.

But as a physician, I know that those bodily systems with which each of us was equipped can be drained by unhealthy attitudes and warped by unwise choices.

As a Christian, I'm convinced that a personal relationship with God can stimulate recovery and help us stay well—in two distinct ways.

First, I believe that a relationship with God provides a firm foundation on which to build those positive attitudes which reduce stress and enable our immune systems to work effectively. Second, I believe that a relationship with God can lead us to make lifestyle choices which improve rather than damage health.

My spiritual secrets are, simply put, practical steps which anyone with faith can take to develop a calm and hope-filled spirit and practical choices which anyone at all can make to develop a lifestyle which promotes good health.

What's Ahead in This Book?

In the next chapters I want to help you understand more about your immune system and how God designed it to protect your health. I want to help you sense how powerfully your outlook—your attitude toward your life—can affect your recovery and promise a lifetime of staying well. You might say I want to give you a scientific basis for confidence in the spiritual secrets I plan to share.

In chapters 3 through 6, I focus on recovery. I want to teach you the attitudes that can stimulate your recovery from even the most serious of human illnesses. And I want to show you step by step how to develop them.

In chapters 7 through 9, I deal with staying well. I

want you to understand how the lifestyle choices you are making even now affect your health. I want to show you simple, easy choices you can make today that will make you more vigorous and make your life more fulfilling.

Throughout the book, I'll simply talk with you as I talk with my own patients, trying not to preach, but honestly sharing those things of which I've become convinced through decades of medical practice and many hours of careful study.

You don't have to follow my advice.

But I want you to. I want you to take my spiritual secrets to heart and be well!

2

—= The Key to
Good Health =—

I watched Sharon grow up. I was her doctor from the time she was about three or four years of age.

Sharon was a Korean war baby—her father was a sailor and her mother a young lady living in a Pacific port. Soon after they were married, Sharon was born.

Sharon was always an independent child with a strong mind of her own. It was obvious very early that this healthy, active girl was going to be a very attractive, outgoing, and free-spirited young adult.

Sharon married in her late teens. It was a turbulent marriage, and it was my impression that she had married for all the wrong reasons. Before too long, the marriage was over and Sharon was struggling to start her life over again. She told me that she was going to be very careful next time around!

In fact, Sharon's personality did change. She became

much more conservative and much more withdrawn. And marriage number two *was* different—she married for money and security.

You can guess what happened to that marriage.

Then came husbands number three and four.

But with her frantic quest for a successful marriage came depression and unhappiness. With each failure, her unhappiness grew deeper.

What had this to do with her health? As the years moved along, I noticed that the number of times Sharon saw me for physical problems increased markedly. She became much more susceptible to infection and seemed to have lowered resistance to bacteria and viruses. She had changed from a healthy young woman to an infectious cripple, her health complicated by eczema, insomnia, and nervousness. Sharon had pushed herself beyond her body's ability to cope, and through a series of wrong choices had converted herself to a near invalid.

Our Ability to Cope

Each of us is born with a God-given physical system that enables us to be healthy. We were created to be healthy! But like Sharon, we can so stress our systems by our choices and our attitude toward life that we can actually make ourselves ill! And we can put so much strain on our systems that, when we are sick, recovery is delayed.

Here are some of these physical systems I'm talking about.

The Respiratory System: This system supplies oxygen to the body, and works much like a bellows. The diaphragm creates a vacuum in the chest, pulling air in through the nostrils. Dust is filtered out by hair, and the air is carried over the mucous membranes at the back of the nose to be warmed and moistened. The air travels into the lungs through the trachea and bronchi where billions of tiny hairlike projections sweep from the lungs any fine dust which eluded the guards above. In the lungs, carbon dioxide in the blood is exchanged for oxygen then exhaled through the same system. Whenever the carbon dioxide builds up in our blood the hypothalamus gland of the midbrain (where the respiratory center is located) sends stronger and more frequent signals directly to the diaphragm, ordering it to contract and pull oxygen into the lungs.

I'm always amused by folks who worry about Junior's attempt to get his way by holding his breath and turning himself blue. This is caused by a build-up of carbon dioxide in the blood, and he'll pass out when he can't hold his breath voluntarily any more. The automatic systems then take over. Junior, unconscious, will breathe quickly as the system automatically expells the carbon dioxide and replaces it with oxygen. In time Junior will learn that holding his breath isn't an effective way to get attention—as long as Mom and Dad don't let him use this way to manipulate them.

This system, by the way, is directly affected by a particular choice that millions of people have made. It's no secret that cancer of the lung is the number one type of cancer in both men and women. That number one ranking is a direct result of smoking.

But the problem with smoking isn't just that it may cause cancer some years down the road.

I mentioned earlier that the trachea and bronchi are lined with billions of sweepers. Well, one drag of cigarette smoke paralyzes these sweepers and they stop working! After a week of smoking the sweepers begin to disappear. With enough smoke, they are gone altogether. The cells the sweepers grew on become inflamed, forming mucus that's dislodged in a smoker's cough. Plugs of this mucus can be inhaled into the lungs, blocking smaller air passages and even causing pneumonia.

The choice to smoke has an immediate and harmful effect on the respiratory system.

By the way, these sweeper cells begin to reappear about a month after a smoker quits smoking.

The Nervous System: Our traceable nerve pathways make man-made communications systems look primitive. The voluntary nervous system starts from the upper brain, where brain cells called neurons initiate a decision to move a muscle. The impulse passes along nerve filaments, and can be followed through the brain, making several connections (something like a great train switchyard) with other nerves. The impulse then runs down the spinal cord. Finally at the nerve/muscle junction the impulse is discharged to make an entire muscle contract. Our decision to make a move is voluntary. But the response of our nervous system is all automatic.

Another system, called the autonomic nervous system, functions twenty-four hours a day. You can't make your heart beat faster or slower at will. Your heartbeat is under control of this special system. When you're frightened, or when you exercise, the autonomic nervous system sends impulses which tell the heart muscle to beat faster because there is a greater demand for oxygen to be delivered to body cells.

Another example of this is the pupil of the eye. You can't control its size; the pupil opens wider or becomes smaller in response to light. It's autonomous. You have no control over it. Blood vessels contract in response to heat or dilate when it's cold. Tears wash the eye. The stomach and bowels all contract, automatically.

Your dual nervous systems, the voluntary and autonomic, illustrate what I'm suggesting in this chapter. Our autonomic nervous system, over which we have no conscious control, is dramatically affected by worry, tensions, fatigue, and stress. In fact, this is the system that is affected the most by a nervous collapse or "breakdown."

Our mental attitude, our psychological and spiritual state, has a direct impact on our physical health.

In fact, I sometimes think that it's more important to heal on the psychological and spiritual level than on the physical.

When Howard came to me, he was troubled by a very painful ulcer. Under treatment, the ulcer healed, but Howard remained nervous, tired, and disturbed. The ulcer I'd dealt with was only the physical symptom of Howard's psychological and spiritual unhealthiness. Howard was "cured," but he was not really *well*. Howard would be well only when the inner psychological or spiritual condition that had contributed to his ulcer and that had made him an unhappy, deeply distressed man, was cured.

In Howard's case, that inner healing was something I was never able to see.

Some doctors might have been satisfied when the ulcer was gone. But I yearned to see Howard truly well.

There are other systems in our makeup that I might describe, piling up illustration after illustration of the way our attitudes and choices affect our health.

We might look at the digestive system, the cardiovascular system, the liver, the brain, the glandular system that keeps thousands of hormones and chemicals in balance, the reproductive system, and others. Whenever I consider any of these unbelievably complex and complicated systems that keep human beings alive and healthy, I have to pause in wonder.

How vast God's understanding is.

How awesome His powers of design. And how wonderful the care He has shown in constructing us, to keep us not just alive, but healthy and well!

Healthy and Well ══════

Before we go on to look at what doctors realize today is the key system affecting our health, I want to acknowledge one thing you may be wondering about. Everyone does not start off in life with the same health advantages. There are genetic differences—characteristics that we inherit from our parents—that affect our bodily systems.

For instance, we've all heard that cholesterol is bad for your heart. Too much cholesterol can coat the walls of your arteries with fatty material, and predispose you to heart attack or stroke.

But cholesterol isn't just a villain. It's an essential ingredient used by cells to make new membranes. And cholesterol is used in the manufacture of various hormones—including male and female sex hormones! So you don't want to be without cholesterol!

But why is this needed substance a problem for some, and not for others? Well, cholesterol is transported through the body inside packets, known as lipoproteins. These are round balls of cholesterol in a protein coating.

There are two kinds of lipoproteins, known as low-density lipoproteins and high-density lipoproteins. Researchers believe that too much low-density lipoprotein promotes heart disease, while plenty of high-density lipoprotein seems to serve as a protection from coronary disease.

We know that a particular gene (a carrier of hereditary traits from one generation to the next) controls the makeup of a protein called apo B. Apo B coats the low-density lipoproteins that carry the "bad" cholesterol. When a cell needs cholesterol, it makes other substances called receptors, that are then attached to the cells' outer coats. These receptors attract the lipoprotein packets passing by in the bloodstream. And one of the receptors is specifically designed to attract apo B protein!

Researchers now believe that a major cause of excess low-density lipoprotein in the blood—and thus a major cause of cholesterol-related heart problems—is a defect in the normal apo B gene. Many of these lipoprotein packets coated with defective apo B do not respond to the receptor substances, and finally pile up as fatty layers inside the blood vessels.

It's pretty clear that someone with a normal apo B gene has a health edge on a person in whom that gene is defective. It's also clear that a person with that genetic defect needs to watch his or her diet much more carefully, and keep down the level of "bad" cholesterol he or she takes in.

Take another case. Our voluntary nervous system, that complicated network which generates and passes on impulses from the mind to the body, will not work if a chemical known as acetylcholine is absent at the nerve junctions. If that chemical is deficient or absent, a person becomes weak and unable to function. The disease is known as myasthenia gravis. You and I have no control over the presence or absence of that chemical.

So it's true.

In some of us, one of the physical systems that makes for good health will be genetically stronger than the same system in others. In a few cases a genetic factor will even mean the difference between sickness and health. *But in most cases, the genetic differences simply mean we may need to adjust our lifestyle.*

In a very real way, what is important for you and me is to make the most of the potential with which we were born. We need to make the choices, and live the kind of lives, that keep our systems functioning up to their potentials.

For a person with a defective apo B gene, that choice may well be to limit intake of cholesterol.

But there are some choices that can destroy health no matter how strong our physical systems may be. And there are other choices that can lead to an experience of vibrant good health, within the limits of our individual genetic makeup, all the time!

But before we look at those crucial choices, let's glance at one other system that constantly functions in our bodies—a system acknowledged today to be the most important health system of all.

Your Immune System

In the past twenty-five years medical science has discovered another system that we now realize plays the key role in our wellness. In fact, to even talk about health today without mentioning this very complex and efficient system would be totally absurd. This is our immune system.

Our immune system is a complex and alert defense network: our shield against illness. Without its protection, we couldn't last a week. Without its protection, some virus or bacteria would invade and kill. Many doctors believe that we have cancer cells in us all the time, and that we survive only because of our immune system's active anticancer defenses.

What at one time was considered a rather dull cell called a lymphocyte has been found to be the key to our immune system. The cell is formed in the marrow of the bones and in the liver, and can actually clone (or duplicate) itself in lymph nodes as it circulates in the blood. Lymphocytes come in different sizes, and usually are round, with a solitary nucleus. The lymphocyte has been found to have the capacity to program itself—almost to the point of thinking for itself. In fact, scientists have called it a "floating brain."

When the body is invaded by a virus, for instance, lymphocytes rush through the circulation system to alert the tissues to what's coming and how to guard against it. Another type of lymphocyte, called a macrophage, tries to surround the viruses and destroy them. Other lymphocytes assume different roles to rid the body of the intruder and maintain wellness.

One of the amazing characteristics of these cells is that they are able to produce minute quantities of substances as a specific defense against the invaders, whether they be bacteria, viruses, or cancer cells. These defense substances are known as lymphokines, and lymphokines are the focus of much current research to solve the problem of cancer and AIDS. At present, the AIDS virus overpowers the lymphokines, and makes the immune system helpless.

At the moment, our research is focused on isolating and duplicating lymphokines. As I write, interleukin 1 and 2 are being used experimentally in cancer treatment—with very impressive results! The antibody programmed to attack the specific cancer target is coated with a lymphokine such as interleukin 2. In effect that antibody becomes a magic bullet, set to attack the specific disease. Right now one lymphokine is being successfully used to attack a cancer tumor and literally dissolve it! Surely we can expect many more lymphokines to be discovered.

Lymphokines are very powerful and quite toxic, so they must be used carefully. It will be a few more years before they can be used extensively. But this is the most exciting breakthrough that's come for some time, because it attacks cancer in an entirely new way. We've previously depended on surgery, radiation, and chemotherapy. Now we use the body's own immune defenses, and if the body cannot produce enough of an interleukin, we may be able to make it in the laboratory and make up the deficit!

I could go on reciting fascinating facts about our immune system. But let me underline my point. The important and fascinating thing is that *good physical health is now understood to depend on a healthy, active immune system,* along with the cooperative, interacting functions of our other physical systems.

And *we know that an active, strong immune system is far more than a matter of medical mechanics!*

In fact, more than any other system, the active normal functioning of our immune system hinges on our basic outlook on life and on the lifestyle choices that you and I make.

Body, Soul, and Spirit ════════════

The other day I picked up a newspaper headlining what it called the "mind-over-illness controversy." The writer quoted a *New England Journal of Medicine* article which argued that there was no relationship between attitude and survival or recurrence of cancer in 359 cancer patients.

It's unfortunate that the phrase "mind-body" has been associated with the kind of healing that I'm writing about in this book, as if someone could by conscious effort exercise control over the complex systems automatically at work within our bodies. Mind over matter, or the notion that if you refuse to believe you're sick, you won't be sick, isn't involved at all. What is involved, and what doctors acknowledge, is that there is a direct relationship between our mental or psychological state and how well our bodily systems function. To be even more specific, *there is a growing conviction in the medical community that links do exist between our mind, or psychological state, and the immune system.*

Immunology Today, a scholarly journal, cites "much evidence" from developments in a field called psychoimmunology. The fact is that researchers have been able to define some of the specific mechanisms on a cellular and molecular level that serve as a link between the human mind and the immune system!

I've been a doctor far too long and worked with far

too many patients to have any doubt that physical well-being is intimately linked with our psychological and our spiritual state.

That's why I shared the story of Sharon at the beginning of this chapter. Sharon became chronically ill from the stress of her unwise choices. Her unhappiness threw her immune and other systems out of balance. She quite literally made herself sick!

Millions of other people are making themselves sick in exactly the same way because they lack the perspective on life provided by faith, and because they lack the inner strength and security that might be theirs through a personal relationship with a Supreme Being.

Let me give just one example of what I mean by perspective on life—something we'll look at more carefully later. Dr. F. Paul Kosbab, a native of Berlin, Germany, describes one way that Christian faith moves us toward health and wellness:

> The frustration that many people are feeling is that of not having certain *luxuries* that others have. They feel stress because they are working for possessions. To be released from stress, a person needs to develop an internal sense of happiness which is not dependent solely on possessions. And that is a spiritual element. The best things in life are still free—such as being alive, breathing, being free of pain, being able to look at the sunshine and the blue sky. Being able to enjoy our children. That's not to say that God doesn't want us to have material things. But the pursuit of possessions must be in a proper perspective.*

The person whose Christian values are reflected in his or her outlook on life may have far less unhealthy pressures and stress, and put far less strain on his or her immune system.

Abundant Life, Vol. 36, December 1982, pp. 18–19.

I'm convinced that physical health and wellness are ours when our bodies' systems function as God designed them to function. And I am absolutely sure that the way your body's systems function depends in turn on your psychological and spiritual state.

The choices you make and the values you choose to live by can keep your immune and other systems healthy. A trusting, confident, and hopeful attitude, rooted in your faith, will do more than help you *stay* well. That kind of faith will also help you *get* well!

Your attitude can even make the difference in your recovering from a life-threatening illness like cancer!

Does this mean that a person with a strong faith will never be sick, or is guaranteed healing if a serious illness strikes? Not at all. But a person with a strong Christian faith has many natural advantages, as well as the supernatural advantage of a personal relationship with our God of miracles.

Let's go back a minute.

One of the symptoms of psychological and spiritual imbalance is extreme stress. Under stress we begin to feel anxious and insecure. When stress is chronic, as in Sharon's case, the immune and other systems are thrown out of balance. You ache in your upper back and neck, you get headaches, nausea, dry mouth, cramps, dizziness, any of a number of symptoms. Why? Because thousands of hormones, enzymes, and chemicals are out of balance. And when that happens, you are a prime candidate for something disastrous to move in!

So what's the solution? The answer is both simple and difficult. The simple part is, you've got to change *inside*. The hard part is—how?

As a doctor, I never give a person the advice to "just shape up, and pull yourself together." That's bad advice, because it is impossible for a person to change his own sensitive, insecure self. We need something or someone from outside to rescue us from ourselves.

There are many roads to the stressed situation in which your immune and other systems are thrown out of balance. It can be a tragedy, the loss of a spouse, a bad marriage, wrong choices, and so forth. But when these lead to a trauma of the spirit, or a sick spirit, that in turn is almost sure to lead to a sick body.

No wonder most illness is now seen as coming from within rather than from without! You don't need to "catch" germs from someone else. All you need is for your immune system to be so depressed it can't fight the germs or viruses already in your body.

I believe that for many of us the way back to health begins when we believe in the living God who cares. You can't change yourself, or heal your own sick spirit, but He can. As we learn to trust Jesus, and surrender ourselves to Him, the panic is arrested. His Spirit speaks to your spirit, quieting and bringing inner peace. The journey back to health may not be rapid; it seldom happens overnight. But as God's Spirit works within to bring quiet and peace, our systems can find their balance points again and healing can take place.

Some Christians who have never experienced that very intimate and personal relationship of living in fellowship with God may have missed this inner peace. As a result they too may not be well, or may be fighting a losing battle against disease. Discovering the deeper meaning of relationship with Christ can also set such persons on the road to renewed health.

As I said, belief in Jesus does not guarantee physical health. It won't change the gene that controls your apo B, and it may not stimulate production of acetylcholine, the villain in myasthenia gravis. But faith does provide inner strength. Trust in a living God brings us that peace of mind—a healthy spirit and healthy soul—so vital if our immune system is to function as God intends.

This is one of the major things I try to teach my patients—how to draw on a relationship with Jesus to promote healing, and keep them well. And I also try to teach them the moral and health choices they need to make to keep bodily systems functioning up to their full potential.

When I'm able to treat the body, the soul, *and* the spirit of my patients, then and only then am I doing all I can do as a physician and healer of men.

So let me tell you again what's ahead for you in this book. First, I'm going to share with you the same spiritual secrets of vital good health that I've shared with the men and women who've come to my office these past forty years. I'm going to take you, step by step, through the process of developing a faith that can help restore the balance of your immune system and promote your healing.

In teaching you this I'm not expressing doubt that God sometimes works miracles of healing. In fact, I consider the human body and the complex systems I've touched on here to be constant miracles. Only by God's creative and sustaining touch could such amazing processes go on continually. What I am convinced of is that God *typically* heals through the miraculous "normal" processes He has built into our bodies, hearts, and minds.

My spiritual secrets of vital good health are simply ways to help you live in touch and in harmony with our miracle-working God, opening up your heart and life to His transforming power. As you live in fellowship with God and with His principles, you will experience the benefits of that vital good health He is eager to give.

Part I

Spiritual Secrets
of Recovery

3

Why Me, God?

I always dreaded hearing Mr. Kay in my waiting room. I could always tell he was there by the critical, judgmental tone I heard as the sound of his voice filtered into my examining rooms.

Mr. Kay was an older gentleman who wore his religion on his sleeve. He would hobble into my office with a bundle of tracts, and immediately start talking with any other patients waiting to see me. If someone there had a cough, or rough breathing, he was quick to point out that they wouldn't be sick if they didn't smoke. According to Mr. Kay, these people were getting just what they deserved!

He'd ask people about their religious beliefs, and if they didn't believe exactly as he did, Mr. Kay would tell them they were going to hell. What's more, he would assure them they were going to suffer in this world, too, because God had rejected them.

"God has a people He blesses," Mr. Kay was fond of saying. And he seemed to take delight in letting my patients know that they weren't in that blessed company!

Finally I had to tell him to quit talking to the other patients in my office.

But what was so interesting to me was that Mr. Kay was one of the most insecure people I ever met. He became alarmed over slight symptoms which any well-balanced person would ignore. He often would phone me, going into great detail over insignificant things that he had magnified. Mr. Kay's fears had cut his ability to handle stress to near zero, and he seemed to make no attempt to improve his position.

In fact, he didn't even recognize his position. Mr. Kay claimed to have great faith in God, and what God would do for him. But his actions didn't match his words.

As a result of his insecurity he was always sick, down with repeated colds, flu, and a variety of illusive body aches and pains. Insomnia was also one of his prominent symptoms.

One Saturday morning Mr. Kay called me at home and started another recital of complaints. Finally he said, "Why does God do this to me? I have been a good man, and have always kept the commandments. Why does He do this to me?"

Now that was a leading question!

As sternly as I could, I told Mr. Kay that he was blaming God for something in which He was not involved. By his own choice, Mr. Kay had allowed himself to be consumed with self-pity. His own insecurity had created a climate in which it was almost impossible for him to feel well.

Mr. Kay demonstrates what happens to people every day. Did you know that 90 percent of the people who complain of fatigue yet have no abnormal physical or laboratory findings at the time of examination are suffering from a psychological disarray?

One of the most common complaints in the doctor's office is, "Doctor, I'm tired," or "I just don't feel like doing anything." Each one who comes to the doctor with this complaint thinks he has something wrong that explains the fatigue. Mr. Michael Halberstam, of George Washington University in Washington, D.C., conducted an experiment, exploring the causes of fatigue with colleagues. He found that only one in thirty-eight patients had any organic problem that accounted for the tiredness! His point was that, in the great majority of cases, people with this single complaint are tired as a result of psychological problems. To correct the symptom, treatment must be directed toward the psyche.*

It's all right to ask, "Why me, God?" But the real question for Mr. Kay and for many other patients I see isn't "Why am I sick?" but "Why am I so psychologically fragile that I am anxious, nervous, and upset? And what can I do to relieve my insecurity?"

Don't get me wrong. I can understand that agonized first reaction to serious illness. When I was diagnosed as having a serious cancer, my first reaction was just the same. "Why me, God?"

But then, as I thought more about it, I found my question changing. "Why not me, God?"

You and I live in an imperfect world, a world contaminated with all sorts of illnesses and afflictions. I began to ask myself what right I had to suppose that, just because I believed in God, I'd be spared illness or even premature death.

During my medical practice I've witnessed all sorts of responses to affliction, from total denial and anger toward God to gracious acceptance. I'm always amazed at the number of professing Christians who suppose they should be exempt from the hard things in this world

---

*"Fatigue," *Current Diagnosis Six.* Howard F. Conn and Rex B. Conn, Jr., eds. (Philadelphia: W. B. Saunders Co., 1980), 50–53.

because they are believers. To them, God is an insurance policy, and to suppose that faith in Him does not make them immune to hardship seems a lack of trust.

Well, it just doesn't work that way. Nowhere in Scripture do I see that Christians are spared the problems common to this world. The apostle Paul didn't seem to expect immunity for Epaphroditus (Phil. 2:25–27), or even for himself (2 Cor. 12:7–10). I have to agree with Peter, and I tell my Christian patients, "Dear friends, do not be surprised at the painful trial you are suffering, as though something strange were happening to you" (1 Peter 4:12).

But being a Christian does make a difference. A secure faith in God gives us the grace and strength to face our difficulties with hope and peace. And, just as Mr. Kay's insecure faith contributed to making him constantly ill, so a secure faith can contribute to keeping us well—and making us well again when serious illness strikes.

So let's go back to a question I asked earlier in connection with Mr. Kay. What makes us so psychologically fragile that we are anxious, nervous, and in fact contributors to our own illnesses? And what can we do to correct our insecurity? What can we do to claim God's promise of inner rest?

God of Love ════════════

One attitude which baffles me is something I see in far more patients than you might imagine. It's the attitude that their illness is punishment. God is "getting them" for something terrible they've done.

I've seen this attitude in Christians and non-Christians alike. It's called guilt.

Feelings of guilt lead directly and rapidly to depression. You can see why. Once a person has accepted the notion that God is angry at him, what follows is depression, loneliness, and despair. A guilt-ridden person is filled with doubts, anxiety, insecurity, and a full complement of other emotions that retard healing. A person like this is in no position to combat disease.

Dora felt just this way when she learned that she needed a mastectomy. Her cancer was well established, and I had to remove her breast.

Dora not only felt abandoned by God, but she was also terrified that her husband would reject her, too. Dora and her husband had enjoyed a good marriage, and a particularly good sex life. Now Dora was sure that her husband would no longer want her sexually.

Dora became extremely depressed, sinking deeper and deeper into despair, unwilling to talk with anyone about her feelings.

But Dora's husband didn't respond as she had feared. All during her illness and recovery, Jim was attentive and loving. I've seldom seen a more supportive husband. In fact, the illness seemed only to draw Jim and Dora closer. And then Dora discovered that Jim still wanted her as much, or perhaps even more, than before.

I asked Jim and Dora to join me on my regular Seattle radio program. She told about her mastectomy and her fears. And then she said, "I'd never want to go through it again. But I wouldn't have missed my sickness for anything. It brought us so much closer together."

That was just what I'd wanted my listeners to hear. Dora's sickness wasn't something that she enjoyed. None of us welcome the pain of suffering. But her sickness was not an evil. Instead, it was just a mixed good. God hadn't been punishing Dora. Instead He had used Dora's illness to draw her and Jim closer together. God used the illness to make a good marriage even better.

I know that my own cancer brought me personal blessings, too. I had time to stop and reevaluate my life. I looked again at my priorities. And I began to notice little things I'd overlooked—little things that make life rich and beautiful, like sunset over the lake, the ripples on the water, the markings on the ducks that paddle by my dock. No, I didn't enjoy my cancer. I didn't get a great deal of pleasure out of the surgery, chemotherapy, or radiation. But the experience deepened my faith in God and blessed me with a renewed sensitivity to the beauty of things I'd been too busy to enjoy. My cancer wasn't God's punishment. It was an instrument of growth and blessing. God constantly showed His love during the whole time I was sick. As I was able to sense His love, I knew an inner peace and confidence that I am sure made the difference in the complete recovery I've enjoyed.

Feelings of guilt, and the fear that God is punishing us, are the enemies of healing. We can see the impact of guilt on the psyche in one of David's most significant psalms. Psalm 32 graphically describes what happens within us:

> When I kept silent,
>   my bones wasted away
>   through my groaning all day long.
> For day and night
>   your hand was heavy upon me;
> My strength was sapped
>   as in the heat of summer (Ps. 32:3, 4).

I've seen these exact symptoms in hundreds of patients. In fact, a great majority of the people who came to me for help had an element of psychological deficit that crippled them to varying degrees. I could hardly believe it at first as I watched the parade of anxious and insecure people pass through my offices. Feeling weak and helpless and drained of strength, these people lacked the inner spiritual resources so essential in combating disease.

But in his psalm David doesn't remain weak and helpless. His psalm goes on:

> Then I acknowledged my sin to you
>   and did not cover up my iniquity.
> I said, "I will confess
>   my transgressions to the Lord"—
> and you forgave
>   the guilt of my sin (Ps. 32:5).

David consciously turned *to* the Lord, and not only acknowledged his sins but also recognized a forgiving God.

This is what always shocks me so much when I see Christians full of symptoms like David's, doubt and anxiety and the torment of guilt. Those feelings of guilt are justified, because my patients *are* guilty. We're all guilty! But Jesus came to die for us. Our sin and guilt have been erased by the cross, and we don't have to carry that guilt around with us all the time.

We don't have to feel afraid. We don't have to feel rejected. We don't have to feel helpless. In spite of our weaknesses and failings, God loves us and has chosen to make us members of His family.

One of the most powerful New Testament passages affirms God's love:

> At just the right time, when we were still powerless, Christ died for the ungodly. Very rarely will anyone die for a righteous man, though for a good man someone might possibly dare to die. But God demonstrates his own love for us in this: While we were still sinners, Christ died for us.
>
> Since we have now been justified by his blood, how much more shall we be saved from God's wrath through him! For if, when we were God's enemies, we were reconciled to him through the death of his Son, how much more, having been reconciled, shall we be saved through his life! (Rom. 5:6–10).

We have compelling evidence of God's love for us in Jesus—such compelling evidence that we can only agree with the apostle Paul that "in all things God works for the good of those who love him" (Rom. 8:28). The evidence?

> He who did not spare his own Son, but gave him up for us all—how will he not also, along with him, graciously give us all things? . . . Who shall separate us from the love of Christ? Shall trouble or hardship or persecution or famine or nakedness or danger or sword? . . . No, in all these things we are more than conquerors through him who loved us (Rom. 8:32–37).

When we approach a sickness from the stance of conquerors, sure that God loves us and is with us, the peace and confidence that comes enables all our physical systems to function at their peak.

Now, I'm not saying that a Christian should never be afraid, or never feel down. Every human being is vulnerable to depression. All of us will have moments of anxiety under stress. What I am saying is that Christians need not be dominated by their feelings. Faith calls on us to turn our attention from our feelings to God, and to affirm the good news of the gospel.

No matter how I feel right now, I know because of Jesus that God loves me.

No matter how I feel right now, I know because of Jesus that God is for me.

No matter how I feel right now, I know because of Jesus that I have hope and a future.

As we focus on the solid reality of our faith, those feelings of insecurity and anxiety will change. As we focus on the reality of Jesus and as that strength grows in our hearts, we *will* know peace. And with peace we're released from the psychological enemies of healing. With inner spiritual peace our bodily systems are free to function as God intended, and to make us well.

I've been Roy's doctor for many years. Roy's a super salesman, driven almost beyond his capacity. Partly because he can't live up to his own expectations, this intense man imagines himself to be sick much of the time. He continually examines himself, and hurries to me whenever he finds anything out of the ordinary. As his doctor, I often have to convince him that nothing is wrong with him. Roy continues to be a top salesperson, but he pays a price for the stress of his work in insecurity about his health.

Roy is an active Christian, and there's no doubt of his sincerity. How can he be an active Christian and still be so anxious? Well, like most of us, Roy doesn't have it all together. But I am sure that without his faith, Roy wouldn't make it at all.

Mary, at fifty-five, is one of the most secure people I've ever known. She married her high school sweetheart, and they worked hard together for years. Shortly after they retired, Mary developed some bowel problems, and she came to me.

I've known Mary as a friend for years—in fact, I grew up with her. And we always kept in touch. Now Mary was in trouble and needed help. She had a cancer of the large bowel.

Mary took the news like the champ she is. I assisted my partner in the operation and monitored her postoperative care. When Mary developed an obstruction, I had to tell her she needed to be operated on again.

Doctors don't usually like to operate on people close to us. But my partner had gone out of town and Mary convinced me she would feel more secure if I did the surgery. Her courage in the time of crisis really impressed me. She faced the new surgery as she had the first, with confidence and total peace.

Mary had an amazingly rapid recovery, and I always accuse her of a superhuman effort just to make me look good. She knew how worried I was about her. But her faith never wavered, and Mary showed not one bit of anxiety or tension.

Roy and Mary both have a real faith in God. And that faith has made a difference in each of their lives. Faith enables Roy to stand the pressures of his work, even though those pressures show up in insecurity about his health. And faith gave Mary an inner peace that I am convinced led to her full recovery.

When we anchor our lives in the assurance that God accepts us, we have a defense against the very natural fears and doubts that stress our bodily systems and work against our recovery.

In Touch

I've already told you that most of the people who come to me for help have an element of psychological disarray that cripples them to a varying degree.

At first I couldn't believe it. Where did this parade of anxieties and insecurities come from? And how could I help?

After getting to know people's individual needs, I now try to start everyone on a routine I follow myself. Included in the routine is something I call "Lone Time."

Just as our physical body needs exercise to keep fit, our spiritual capacities need to be exercised, too. Lone Time is dedicated to maintaining a relationship with God, to avoiding the separation which leads to spiritual starvation and ineffectiveness. I've found, too, that Lone Time creates and maintains a sense of security, and increases our sense of worth and value. I'm convinced that a healthy relationship with our Creator is the key to success as individuals and certainly the key to vital good health.

What do I do for my own Lone Time, and what do I advise my patients?

(1) Set a time when you can be alone and uninterrupted. It needn't be a long time—just fifteen minutes

will do. But it must be a time when you can be quiet and alone.

(2) Begin that time by asking, "Lord, what do You have in store for me today?" Then be quiet, relax, and control your thoughts so that they do not drift off into the problems of the day.

(3) Spend a few minutes reading something inspirational. Right now I'm reading an excellent book, a paraphrase of the Psalms called *Psalms Now,* by Leslie Brandt. My reading reminds me that I am special to God, and I can depend on Him. What I choose to read needs to be something that reminds me of the proper relationship between God and me, something that gives me confidence that my Creator is living, that He cares, and that He has a plan for me. With my relationship with God reaffirmed, I can face the problems of the day without fear or timidity. My spirit has been nurtured, and the psychological symptoms of stress begin to disappear.

(4) After reading the words of inspiration, I become quiet again. I commune with my Creator by talking with Him. I tell my patients that they can talk with God just as they would talk with their best friend, because God *is* their best Friend. So many people tell me, "I can't do that. I wouldn't know what to say." My reply is, "Did you have trouble talking to your daddy when you were two years old?" A smile appears, and it's amazing how many people see God in the proper light for the first time. We needn't fear God. He is our Father, our Daddy, and He loves us.

I encourage all my patients to start the day with a Lone Time. I want them to begin the day with a sense of God's acceptance and His love. I want them to begin their day with confidence and in peace.

Margaret was middle-aged when she came to see me as a patient. She was working in a laundry as a steam presser. As I took her history, it was obvious she had

Passages for Lone Time

When you feel . . .   *Turn to* . . .

Angry	Ps. 86:15; Prov. 17:13; Eph. 4:26–27; James 1:19–20; Phil. 2:3.
Anxious	Exod. 33:14; Num. 6:24–26; 1 Chron. 29:11; Ps. 69:33, 85:8; Isa. 26:3, 32:17; Rom. 5:1–2; 2 Cor. 9:10–11; Phil. 4:19; Col. 3:15.
Confused	Ps. 16:7, 32:8, 86:11; Jer. 31:9; John 8:12; Phil. 1:9–10; James 1:5.
Dejected	Ps. 73:25–26, 86:5; Jer. 24:7, 29:13; Rom. 8:26–27; Heb. 4:15–16.
Depressed	Exod. 33:19; Deut. 31:9; Ps. 42:11, 119:76; Isa. 35:10, 54:8; Jer. 31:13.
Despairing	Ps. 46:1, 100:5, 119:116; Isa. 34:16, 40:29; Jer. 32:17; Hag. 2:4; Eph. 1:18; 2 Thess. 3:3; Heb. 10:35; James 1:12.
Fearful	Deut. 1:17, 7:21; Neh. 4:14; 1 Chron. 16:25–26; Isa. 35:4, 41:10; Jer. 15:20; Phil. 4:9; 1 Peter 3:14–16.
Guilty	2 Sam. 14:14; Neh. 9:17; Ps. 32:2, 5, 103:1–4, 130:3–4; Isa. 43:25, 55:7; Jer. 3:12, 33:8; Dan. 9:9; Mic. 7:18–19; John 3:18; 1 Cor. 6:11; Eph. 3:12; Col. 1:12–14.
Insecure	John 17:11; Eph. 1:17–19, 3:18–19; Phil. 1:9–11; Col. 3:16.
Unloved	Ps. 4:3, 57:3, 89:33; Isa. 43:1, 54:10; Ezek. 34:31, 36:9; Mal. 3:17; Matt. 10:30–31; John 3:16.
Weak	1 Chron. 16:11; Ps. 37:10–11, 55:18, 62:11, 72:13, 142:3, 147:6; Isa. 57:15; Jer. 10:6; Hab. 3:19; 2 Cor. 12:9; Eph. 3:16.

more than the usual number of complaints. And they didn't fit into any pattern of organic disease.

The more I talked with Margaret, the more obvious it was that she was a very unstable person and that her symptoms were rooted in her psychological state. Surprisingly, Margaret realized her problem even though her symptoms were so very real to her.

I even trumped up some other ridiculous symptoms, and after some suggestion, Margaret adopted them as her own!

Margaret, of course, really was physically sick. She was subject to many infections, and had been diagnosed with malignancies. But her problems were far deeper than the physical symptoms I have treated.

I saw Margaret for more than fifteen years, and she continued to get worse. She would go to psychiatrists, but she always ended up coming back to me, claiming she got more help talking to me than she did to a psychiatrist. That's not unusual, of course. A psychologically dependent person will usually attach to someone or something. Margaret attached to me. But she was someone I simply could not help.

I talked with Margaret many times and often explained at length her only hope for relief. Margaret openly blamed God for her misery; she truly was (and still is) miserable. I told her that the God she blamed for her trouble is the only One who can liberate her. But Margaret was unwilling to change, unable to reach out to enjoy the freedom the gospel can offer.

They've all passed through my office these past forty years. The Mr. Kays, whose aggressive talk of God masks inner insecurity and fears. The Margarets, who refuse to look for liberation to a God they blame for all their ills. The Roys, who trust God but still need reassurance. And the Marys, whose deep faith is expressed in confidence and calm in any crisis.

I've been their physician and friend, and as I've
shared their lives I have become more and more convinced that the foundation for recovery from our physical ills is found in a personal relationship with God.

That relationship begins when we come to see God as
He really is, the God of love who loves us so much He
was willing to give His only Son that we might find
forgiveness and new life through Him.

But many Christians miss the full benefits of their
faith by failing to grow in their relationship with the
Lord. That's why Lone Time is so important. As we take
the time to be alone with the Lord, as we focus on who
He is and the greatness of His love for us, His Spirit
speaks to our spirits and He brings us peace. As Jesus
said, "Peace I leave with you; my peace I give you. I do
not give to you as the world gives. Do not let your hearts
be troubled and do not be afraid" (John 14:27).

In Jesus we find peace.

As we claim His peace, our spirits are healed, our
hearts find rest, and the wonderful systems that God
created in our bodies are released to bring us wholeness
and health.

4

Medical Care

When I went into the hospital for my cancer operation, I got a patient's eye view of modern medical care.

From the moment I hit the admitting room, I was depersonalized.

First I was asked all sorts of intimate questions by a person I didn't know. Then I was strapped with a wristband for "identity" (I already knew who I was). Then I had to give up my wallet for "safe keeping," and I was escorted to the lab for routine blood and urine tests.

The blood was easy enough. But did they really need that much?

Then came the request for urine. "But I just went."

"Well, squeeze out a little."

That's easy for them to say. But did you ever try to squeeze out just a little in a strange place, with strange noises, and in a threatening environment?

By this time, even though I'm a doctor and familiar with hospitals, I was beginning to feel insecure and anything but comfortable.

Then I was given a personal packet to take to my room. It consisted of a plastic washpan, a toothbrush, toothpaste, and an emesis basin. (That's a little threatening by itself.) And amidst it all was a little card that read, "Welcome."

In my room I was given a flimsy gown that fit backwards, and was then told to surrender all my clothes.

"*All* my clothes?"

"Yes."

It was only three in the afternoon, much too early to go to bed. But I went to bed. The strange, impersonal room filled with strange odors was hardly a comfort.

About a half hour later someone came with a wheelchair. I asked, "What's that for?"

"You're going to x-ray."

"I can walk."

"No, the orders are for you to go in a wheelchair."

That seemed strange. I walked in, but here they were telling me I couldn't walk any more. I was beginning to wonder if hospital life was for me.

The x-ray department was a regular beehive of activity, so I was left sitting in the hallway dressed in nothing but a brief, open-back gown, with slippers on my cold feet and a blanket over my lap.

After what seemed an eternity, I was finally x-rayed and wheeled back to my room for supper. What a supper! Well, I wasn't all that hungry anyway.

Then I was visited by a doctor who said he's my anesthesiologist, and had just stopped by to ask me some questions. He was pleasant, but obviously busy, and he didn't want to talk very long. He listened to my heart, examined my chart, and left as abruptly as he came.

It didn't take me long to realize that my chart was far

more important to the hospital staff than I was. I spent a restless night.

Early the next morning, I was placed on a cart and wheeled down to the operating room. Again I was left in a hallway, like a plane holding on the runway before takeoff. Eventually I was taken to the operating room, and greeted by the doctor who had visited me the day before. At least, that's who he said he was. I could only see his eyes—the rest of him was covered with the pale green of his surgical hat, mask, shirt, and pants. As the anesthesiologist began his work, I felt myself slipping into unconsciousness.

Strange voices pulled me out of a deep sleep, and I found myself in the recovery room surrounded by even more people I didn't know. One of them gave me a painkiller, and I was extremely grateful. It not only made my pain go away, but all my apprehensions with it.

I noticed that my chart went everywhere with me, and people had a tendency to leaf through it and then write something on it.

My mouth was dry, and I had no water. Finally someone gave me a drink.

Then I was told that I had to try to urinate, but I couldn't. An aide came in and told me to try harder. Well, I knew that wasn't going to work, and when it didn't she called a nurse. This was another person whom I was seeing for the first time. She didn't have time to talk to me, but began writing in that chart. Then she told me in a kind but positive way to stand up. She carefully helped me get my feet to the floor, and then she told me not to worry—she'd steady me while I urinated.

How could I do anything with a nurse holding me up? That was psychologically and physiologically impossible. I said, "I don't think I really need to go just yet."

When she left, I got out of bed and limped to the

bathroom. This time I was really motivated! I beat the
system. And it didn't even get on my chart.

But I didn't have the last word. In a while the nurse
came back, and said that if I didn't go of my own accord,
I would have to be catheterized. I made my confession,
which didn't make her too happy.

I resolved then to get out as soon as possible.

I spent three days in the hospital, and had good scientific care. But I had poor personal care. It's almost impossible to have good personal care in our present
system.

What's Happened to Personal Care? ════════

In my forty years in medicine I've witnessed the evolution of the modern hospital, with all its new technology and the wonderful things we can now do because
of scientific advancements. But I've also witnessed—
and experienced!—the depersonalization of the patient.

There was a day when the patient was the center of
the hospital world, and every effort was made to make
him or her feel comfortable and at ease. There was time
then for the nurse to treat the patient with obvious caring. I remember when each patient got a back rub, and
was prepared for the night by the nurse. There was time
then for communication, and the nurse's touch had powerful healing properties. Patients responded to that
kind of attention, and we have overwhelming research
evidence that personalized patient care actually expe-
dites healing and recovery. Unfortunately, because of a
shift in priorities to administration, there's a real tension between hospital administrators and the people
who deliver patient care. It's reached a point where the
chart has become so important that the nurse has pre-
cious little time with the patient.

There is nothing in the present system that ministers

to the inner person. Yet medicine must at its very heart be a ministry and not a profession.

Now, I've not shared this with you to frighten you, or to criticize the medical community. I'm so grateful for the technological advances that enable medical people to deal with illnesses we couldn't touch forty, or even twenty, years ago. And I'm grateful for the growing emphasis in medical schools on the need to minister lovingly to patients as whole persons. I also have some very practical suggestions for you, if you are ever a patient, as you select and work with your medical care people. These suggestions can make a real difference in your recovery.

But you need to understand something of what's happened in medicine these past forty years, and why the suggestions I'm going to make are so important.

Since World War II, the practice of medicine has gone through a dramatic evolution. No longer do Americans see the neighborhood doctor, who was not only a health adviser but also a friend, comforter, and in some cases even a priest. There was a bond then between the patient and the doctor that gave each family a sense of security. The doctor offered more than medical advice and help.

Technology then was in its infancy, and the methods of treatment used in the forties seem quite primitive to us now. But the patients received an element of support and personal attention lacking in the present method of health care delivery.

The irony is that the curative and preventive methods of the past were adequate or even superior for 75 percent of the patients who sought advice for their health problems. The close doctor-patient relationship was very important to the patient's well-being. But little by little, this closeness has been eroded.

During the evolution of high technology, the general practitioner found himself in an increasingly awkward position. His status in the medical community was continually being downgraded by a trend toward specialization, an idea which seemed very attractive to the younger doctor. He would no longer be a suburban family practitioner, but rather an *authority* in a smaller branch of medicine. Little by little the doctor ceased to be the family counselor or priest. He might retain his friendly relationship with the family, but on a limited basis. There was no time to go to the house, to share a cup of coffee or talk about members of the family. The doctor was still friendly, but in a remote sort of way. No longer did the patient feel comfortable discussing intimate family problems which in times past would have cemented the doctor-patient bond. The patient still respected the doctor's knowledge and wisdom, but at the same time the doctor became more of a technician and less of a friend. There was distance between the patient and doctor.

The trend toward specialization had another influence, which is continuing to evolve. Group practice has become the mode. Specialists band together, in groups of anywhere from three to hundreds, under the same roof and under the direction of a staff of administrators. This provides an impressive array of resources for the patient. But the effect is further depersonalization: The sense of comfort that comes from seeing a doctor whom you know and who knows you is lost.

Ironically, that factor—personal relationship and personal support—is vital to recovery from illness.

This hasn't been appreciated until recently. But once again the importance of personal, emotional support is being acknowledged. Presently medical educators have been trying to correct the problem by graduating more family practitioners, seeking to get them to settle in the suburbs and small towns.

We don't want to go back to the technology of the forties. But we do want to find a new, better balance between technology and the personal dimension in medical care.

This growing concern is expressed in many articles, like this one from *Dimensions in Health Service.* The article echoes a warning "that our preoccupation with technology is in danger of overshadowing the 'nonmechanical' aspects of providing care." The article states:

> For instance, consider some of the potentially depersonalizing aspects of sophisticated equipment. Without this equipment, Mr. Jones' condition would be assessed by direct contact with him. A hand would touch him to feel a pulse; now the equipment makes it possible to obtain the information without even entering the room—we engage with the monitor rather than with Mr. Jones.
>
> Modern communications systems, such as the intercoms which replace the traditional call bell, also diminish the necessity for face-to-face contact. The rationale for these systems is to cut "unnecessary visits" to the patient. With the introduction of these systems, communication becomes disembodied. Literally, and figuratively, we lose sight of the significant nonverbal messages.
>
> By replacing our human presence with emotionally nonresponsive pieces of equipment, we are removing one of the most important sources of comfort for the patient. And we are doing this in a circumstance in which the patient's anxiety is already heightened by the mere presence of the machine.*

This article goes on to trace other problems linked with reliance on technology. And it concludes: "It is too easy to neglect or diminish the non-mechanical aspects of care. It is becoming increasingly important that we take every opportunity to humanize our care and to reestablish the priority of the patient over the machine."

---

*E. Durbach and C. MacLeod, "Humanizing Care—Patient vs. Machine," *Dimensions in Health Service* (July 1984).

In some hospitals we *are* seeing attempts to reestablish this priority. The Albert Einstein Medical Center in Philadelphia has launched a HOSPITAL-ity program of training for everyone from doctors to orderlies. Employees take turns playing the part of the patient, and the staff learns to establish a set of rules for patient contact, rules such as, "Introduce yourself. Call people by name. Make eye contact with them. Explain what you are doing." As the importance of caring and its impact on the recovery process becomes more widely understood, hundreds of other facilities are beginning to add similar "guest relations" programs.

I have shared my own experience and the background on what has happened in medicine through technological advances for just one reason: *I want you to understand that feeling comfortable and confident about your medical care is essential to your recovery.*

You need the release that comes from knowing you are in the hands of a competent physician who cares about you as a person. And you need supportive warmth from other health care providers to help you realize that you are important as a person.

Depersonalized health care robs us of a sense of value and worth that is so important during sickness. Sickness itself will tend to threaten any person, and bring doubts and fears. At times like this when we feel so vulnerable we need not only to remember the sustaining power of God; we need to experience caring from the persons around us.

Profiling Your Doctor

Mac was a distinguished man with an outstanding career. He was an FBI agent and became the director of a large FBI district. I don't remember just how he got to me, but I do remember how difficult it was to get a decent history of his medical background. Mac was a very private person. He weighed each question carefully before answering me, and then spoke in a voice just above a whisper.

It was even more difficult to get Mac to come into the office in the first place, but finally he was forced to come. His symptoms were caused by a malignant tumor. Mac had cancer.

At first I'd thought of Mac as stoic and cynical, but I turned out to be wrong. I suppose his lack of transparency was fostered by his work. As Mac learned to trust me, I gradually came to know and appreciate him as a shy, sensitive man of high principles. Mac bonded to me too. Once trust had been established, I was the only medic he would allow to come near him. And as we came to know each other, I always enjoyed talking with him. He was a man of few words, but when he spoke it was with real wisdom.

Mac got well, but after a few years his tumor returned. In time he had to be confined to his home. I went to see him regularly, and during that time I was able to learn his attitude about life and death. More and more he talked to me about the present and the future, and came to enjoy sharing his faith with me.

My experience with Mac illustrates the importance of building up a relationship between doctor and patient over a number of years. Bonding is important. When a person is ill and the doctor has become one of the family, he or she can be made much less anxious just by knowing "my doctor is here."

The other day I reviewed a chart for the grievance committee of the King County Medical Society on which I serve. It was filed by the wife of a very sick man. She complained that he had received poor medical care; no one seemed to know what was going on, and no one was willing to take the time to explain anything to her. As I reviewed the case, I found her husband had nineteen doctors in attendance! It's true, he was in a teaching hospital. Many times a patient gets bounced around like a ping-pong ball in one of these institutions. As I reviewed the chart, I tried to find out just who was in charge. It was impossible! I called three doctors who were assigned to the case, and none had any inkling of what was going on. They remembered seeing the patient. But each declined responsibility: no one was in charge. According to the chart, the man was getting good treatment. But the wife didn't know it, and the patient himself was certainly in the dark. Her grievance was completely valid and real.

It may seem difficult to develop a personal relationship with a doctor in these high-tech days. But it's not impossible. And it's important when sickness comes to have that relationship established!

I know that while I was practicing I did everything I could to encourage a healthy sense of personal relationship with my patients. My office was arranged purposely so that patients waiting in the reception room could see me going in and out of examination areas. I wanted them to know I was busy working and not wasting time. And I wanted them to see progress, so they would know they would be seeing me soon. I also made it a rule not to put a patient in an examining room until I was about to see him. It was much more comfortable in the reception room, and I wanted patients to have access to the warmth of that area.

My staff welcomed every patient personally as he or she entered. They were great at that. In fact, I had patients tell me that they came in partially to see the office personnel. Some of the patients have kept in touch not only with me, but with my staff as well since we all retired.

There's a lot of therapy in that approach. People feel secure and safe just being in the presence of a staff that cares.

If someone needed to be seen, my staff would squeeze

him in somehow that day, not two weeks later. When you hurt, you can't wait two weeks. I screened my staff very carefully, and when I heard one of them be terse, or not really kind to a patient, I had a talk with that individual.

My nurse was with me twenty-three years and the patients loved her. In fact, she knew as much or more about them than I did. I used to chuckle when once in a while I would pick up the phone, when everyone else was busy, and there would be a pause on the other end before the patient would say, "Oh, I really didn't want to talk to you. I wanted to talk to your nurse." Now, that's a great compliment for a great lady named Sully. She cared so much for each patient that they could feel it, and just felt better talking with her.

That really is healing. That's a spiritual dimension too powerful to be measured, and while there is still some of it around today, you've got to look for it.

There are some doctors who think that attachment to a person is not good, and that objectivity is hampered. But no one who has ever been really sick has entertained that thought. No one can feel well, and be suspicious of people and things. *It is vital for a person who hurts to trust. And to trust, you need to know and have confidence in your medical team.*

I've had the joy of seeing the attitudes of people who came to me evolve gradually from doubting suspicion to a faithful trust. I've seen symptoms disappear and frowns change into smiles. Confidence is a radiant thing, and promotes good health and wholeness. There is real healing in the release that comes when you know and trust your doctor, and realize that he is loyal to you as a person and is not just a distant, impersonal technician. As I said, I'm disturbed by the impersonality in much of modern medical practice. Today you have to look harder for doctors who take—or have!—the time to care. But you have one advantage. Today there's a great surplus of doctors. You might say it's a buyer's market. So you can be selective. You don't have to take the first doctor you go to. You can change doctors if you don't feel comfortable with the doctor who is seeing you now. You can look for, and find, a doctor who is interested in you as a whole person. You can find a doctor in whom you have confidence, one to whom you can trust yourself, a doctor who will be God's agent of healing in your life.

How are you going to recognize someone who is the right doctor for you? I've tried to give you an idea of some of the relational dimensions that I feel are important by describing my own office and practice. Now let me give you some specific guidelines.

Dr. Johnson's Guidelines for Choosing a Doctor

Four steps to take:
1. Look for a primary care physician.
2. Gather information on local doctors.
3. Visit doctors' offices.
4. Check medical credentials.

Six qualities to look for:
5. Do your personalities match?
6. Does the doctor communicate well?
7. Does the doctor respect your intelligence?
8. Does the doctor take a careful personal history?
9. Does the doctor display personal discipline?
10. Is the doctor forthright?
11. Is the doctor available?
12. Does the doctor seek second opinions when indicated?

1. *Look for a primary care physician.* It's important to have one doctor who is *your* doctor. Too often these

days people go to one specialist for their ears, another for stomach complaints, and yet another for sprained ankles. Specialists are important in today's complicated medical world. But you should have a primary care physician whom you see regularly. He can advise you when to see a specialist, and what specialist to see.

What kind of doctors provide primary care? Today there are few GPs (general practitioners). But you can find doctors who will care for you as a whole person listed under Family Practitioner or Internist. At times gynecologists will serve as primary care physicians for women, and pediatricians may be primary care physicians for children. These doctors will be concerned with treating *you,* not some specialized illness or injury you may have.

Again, what counts is to have one doctor who is *your* doctor. As you build a relationship with this doctor over a period of time, and he or she comes to know you and your family, your doctor can guide you to any specialists an illness may require.

2. *Gather information on local doctors.* If you're moving, or if you don't have a primary care physician now, how do you find one? There are several sources of information. You can call your county medical society and ask for help. You can chat with friends and new neighbors: What do they know about the doctors in your area? Pharmacists are good sources of information. Who do they consider the best doctors in the area? Another source of information is the local hospital. Get a list of physicians on the staff. Talk with emergency room personnel. Who do they consider the best doctors? If you have doctors who attend your church, check with the specialists about who they consider the best primary care physicians in your area.

As you filter information gathered from sources like these you'll build an impression of the various doctors in your area. You'll eliminate some because of negative impressions. Soon you'll narrow down the list of those you want to consider as your doctor to just a few.

3. *Visit doctors' offices.* You can learn a lot just by a visit to the doctor's office. Is its location satisfactory for you? Is the reception area clean and organized? Does it tend to put you at ease, or is it a cold impersonal area? How does the staff treat you? Can you picture them as being helpful when you need them? This is extremely important for a family practice office. Do not be over-aggressive in this survey. This visit should be short and low key. You are there only to get an impression.

4. *Check medical credentials.* Talk with the office staff. Let them know you're looking for a primary care physician, and ask in a diplomatic way about the doctor's training. Today no one can be aware of every medical discovery: We're in the midst of a true information explosion. You want a doctor who not only is warm and caring, but who is professionally competent as well.

When you've taken these preliminary steps, you need to go to the doctor of your choice for treatment. You may find after a few visits that you want to change doctors. If you feel uncomfortable or uncertain, please do make a change. Go to another doctor on that initial list, or go through the screening process again.

It is vital for recovery that you have a primary care physician whom you trust.

What are some of the personal characteristics of a physician which enhance that sense of trustworthiness? Here are some qualities that I have found are important:

5. *Do your personalities match?* I've always been a casual person. Some patients who came to me felt uncomfortable because I didn't dress in starched whites or maintain what they viewed as proper "professional" distance. Those patients soon left me and found a doctor who fit their notion of what a physician ought to be.

I was glad to see them go. No, I wasn't eager to get rid

of them. But I realized that for me to be effective my patient had to be really comfortable with the kind of person I am. If a patient wasn't comfortable with me, I wanted him or her to find a doctor with whom that comfort factor would exist.

There's really no "right" personality profile for a doctor. What has to be right is the match between the personality of the patient and that of the doctor. If you feel good about your doctor, and comfortable with him or her, then a personality match probably does exist.

6. *Does the doctor communicate well?* Doctors and patients are partners in maintaining health and in speeding recovery. A real partnership means that there needs to be clear communication which flows both ways. Does the doctor take time to explain clearly what he or she has found when examining you? Does he or she explain the results of tests, and discuss treatments prescribed? Do you know why a particular medicine or course of treatment has been recommended? If you feel in the dark about your health, and if your doctor isn't responsive to your questions, then you may need to find another primary care physician. An essential element in trust is the sense that your doctor knows what he or she is doing. And such trust is enhanced by clear, careful communication on his or her part.

7. *Does the doctor respect your intelligence?* Too many of my colleagues tend to become defensive when asked questions. Some will resort to "put-down" retorts that say all too clearly that because you aren't medically trained you simply can't understand. That's wrong. We doctors need to take the complicated and communicate it clearly enough so that patients do understand the basics of their illnesses and their treatment. A doctor who constantly puts down his patients, and shows a lack of respect for their intelligence is unlikely to win the trust so important for continuing good health and recovery.

8. *Does the doctor take a careful personal history?* Today we recommend a physical exam perhaps once every three years up to age fifty, and more often as we grow older. But just as important as the tests associated with a complete physical is the personal history the doctor takes. You probably fill out a preliminary history when you first visit a doctor's office. But your primary care physician will go over this with you carefully. Information about your family members and your lifestyle can sensitize a doctor to various risk factors, and help him or her better interpret your symptoms. It's a positive sign when your doctor takes time with you to develop a careful personal history.

9. *Does the doctor display personal discipline?* For the successful doctor-patient relationship to exist, there must be certain absolutes which are binding to a reasonable degree to both parties. Does the doctor have a reputation for being unreasonably late for his appointments? Is he dependable? This may take a while for you to determine. It would be good to find a doctor whose priorities in life are compatible with your own. Above all, does he seem to be genuinely interested in you and your family?

10. *Is the doctor forthright?* I've known too many doctors who simply can't tell a patient bad news. At times a doctor will keep on prescribing unnecessary tests when he or she knows what's wrong, just to put off a painful confrontation. In all my years of practice, I've never told a patient that he or she is going to die. In the first place, I never know. I've seen far too many unexplained (should we say miraculous?) recoveries for which there were no known medical causes. I can speak of percentages. Something may be fatal within five years for 80 percent of the population. But there are always the 20 percent who recover. And I believe in recovery.

But I also believe in being forthright. If a patient has a serious disease, I believe he or she has a right to know, and to understand what is happening. I always had hope for my patients, and I wanted to communicate that hope. But I did not want to lie or to pretend.

You can trust a doctor who will level with you about an illness, and still treat you with hope and a positive expectation.

11. *Is the doctor available?* Doctors have always been busy, but medicine is a ministry, not an eight-hour-a-day job. If my patients were ill or uncomfortable, I wanted them to come in to see me, or to call me. I knew that I was important to my patient's well-being, and I wanted to be available when I was needed.

The minute a patient believes the doctor is just "in business" and not there to help, something very important in the relationship has been violated. Being available is an important dimension of the doctor-patient relationship, and of the trust so important between them.

12. *Does the doctor seek second opinions when indicated?* One of the greatest resources doctors have is other doctors. Often we will be bothered by some symptom or complaint that just doesn't fit our idea of what's wrong. That's the time a good doctor will seek a second opinion. Actually, it shouldn't be necessary for a patient to ask for a second opinion—the doctor should suggest it. It's not a good sign if your doctor seems to resent a request for a second opinion, or take it as a lack of trust in him or her.

I've included these guidelines on choosing a primary care physician for a single, simple reason. *It's important for your recovery to have a doctor whom you trust, a doctor who is "your" doctor.* The relationship you establish and build over the years with your doctor can make a vital difference in your recovery. That trust and confidence can help to reduce the natural fears and tensions that come with any sickness. The comfort of a caring, trusted doctor can help to bring that calm which releases your immune system to function effectively and help you once again be well.

Hospitalization

I began this chapter with a rather discouraging, though hopefully somewhat humorous, report of my own hospitalization for a cancer operation. While hospital care is becoming more sensitive in some areas, there's much that needs to be done.

What do I recommend when you need to be hospitalized?

First, if you are treated impersonally or gruffly by nursing or other staff, tell your doctor and let him handle the problem. While there are many administrative pressures on hospital employees, there is no excuse for insensitive treatment. If necessary, your doctor may be able to move you to another room or ward.

Second, have as many familiar things with you in the hospital as you are allowed. It's important in a strange and sometimes threatening environment to have the familiar to touch and feel.

But as soon as possible, return home or somewhere you can feel at ease. Set returning home as a goal to achieve, a sign of progress toward getting well.

At home you can wear familiar clothes, while friendly noises and surroundings will put you at ease. It's important to sit in your dining room and eat family food. Even friends are more comfortable visiting in your home. There's enough to deal with in handling a serious disease without doing it in strange territory. More and more patients are going home earlier, and being cared for by visiting nurses. Doctors are even making house calls again. Having a primary care physician who understands the importance of factors like these is a real stimulus to recovery.

In my own case, I didn't want to see friends at first. But I did watch my eating and exercise. In fact, I started riding my bicycle with my wife Genevieve within two weeks after my surgery.

A very important factor in my recovery was my insistence on going to the office about two weeks into my treatment. I didn't go there to work, but being there and seeing the office staff, with everything in place, was a reassuring event that guaranteed my eventual recovery of worth as a person. So getting out, and not allowing your problem to totally change your routine, is important.

All this is part of your medical care. And most of all, the quality of your medical care depends on the choice of a primary care physician whom you trust, and who is willing to treat *you* and not just your physical symptoms.

If you have that doctor whom you trust, his or her sensitivity and the confidence you place in that doctor are factors God can use to help you recover and be well.

5

=A Positive
Outlook=—

Fear is one of the emotions over which we have little or
no control.

Fear is a natural emotion. It prepares the body for
emergencies, although some seem to be faced with a
continual emergency. Mostly, though, people are afraid
of the unknown, the uncontrollable. And when you really think of it, we are surrounded by unknowns and by
the uncontrollable. We are born in mystery, we live in
mystery, and we die in mystery. That's enough to make a
person insecure and fearful right from the start. We
can't predict from one day to the next what is going to
happen, and that feeds our insecurities. In life there are
no guarantees.

Some people are better able to deal with their insecurities than others. These people end up with greater
peace of mind, and with a sense of stability. Others,

particularly when under stress, don't handle their insecurities well at all. In fact, fear leads to worry, and
worry to both stress and distress—a distress which
places strain on the immune system and may lead to
sickness, and which surely will make any recovery much
more difficult.

Recent literature emphasizes the negative impact of
fears and stress on our health. Dr. Alfred Coodley, a
psychiatrist at the University of Southern California
Medical School, says that stress "is the most widespread
medical problem in America today. It's a major con-
tributing factor in 100 percent of diseases." The authors
of the book *Stress, Sanity, and Survival* note that stress
upsets the stomach bringing on ulcers, and boosts blood
pressure, leading to strokes and heart attacks. Another
recent book on stress explains:

> Stress can knock out your immune system. Stress can
> make you sick by wreaking havoc on your immune sys-
> tem, allowing disease to strike much more easily.
> "Stress causes the white blood cells of the immune sys-
> tem to be greatly altered, and this allows sickness to set
> in," says Dr. Robert S. Brown, clinical associate profes-
> sor of psychiatry and behavioral medicine at the Uni-
> versity of Virginia. "What happens is this: in case of
> danger or threat, our bodies pour out hormones, which
> give us additional strength, so we can fight or run
> away. . . . In the civilized world we can't fight or run
> away from our problems. So the extra energy isn't used.
> Instead it remains in our body, harming us by weaken-
> ing our immune system."*

Elmer and Alice Green of the Menninger Clinic are
convinced that medicine has now demonstrated that every change in the physiological state is accompanied by
an appropriate change in the mental and emotional

---

*From *Conquering Stress* (New York: Pocket Books, 1985) p. 29.

state, conscious or unconscious, and conversely, *every change in the mental and emotional state, conscious or unconscious, is accompanied by an appropriate change in the physiological state.*

Human beings are whole: Body, soul and spirit are bound together in a unitary system. If we affect one, we affect the others as well.

Avoiding Stress?

It is a fact of life that no one can really avoid stress. The chart on page 82 was developed to measure the amount of relative stress placed on a person by a variety of experiences. Glance over it, and you'll see that while you may not have every experience listed, you are certain to have not just one but many of them.

We can't avoid the uncertainties of life that cause anxiety and worry in so many persons. *But we need not be destroyed by the stressful experiences that seem to destroy so many. We have a guardian against the harmful effects of stress and the destructive effects of fear.*

I remember one week when two patients, Al and Ben, were diagnosed with the same serious problem: cancer of the right colon, much like the cancer which President Reagan had. Now, that diagnosis of cancer is hard for anyone to take. But when Al heard his diagnosis, he faced it in an upbeat, positive way.

Al was a joy to take care of. Before the surgery the nurses on the floor remarked that he was really a pleasant man, and a good sport in the preparation for surgery.

That preparation isn't easy, because it consists of laxatives and enemas until the bowel is perfectly clean. The success of the operation depends a lot on how the bowel is prepared. The nurses used to laugh at my orders, because I would specify, "Repeat enemas until the results are crystal clear, and I do mean crystal." One nurse used to call me the Crystal Kid.

Al got into the spirit of the whole thing and suggested the nurses call the fire department for bigger hoses. He joked and kidded up until the time he went into surgery. The entire episode was pleasant for everyone involved, including Al.

The surgery went well and Al went off to the recovery room. Sure, when he was coming out of the anesthetic he was uncomfortable, and he was given medication to relieve his pain. But again Al did what the nurses told him, and he returned to his room in good condition.

His postoperative course was smooth. In those days we used blow-up balloons to make the patients breathe. Al made a game out of it, going for the all-time hospital record. He had fun when he could.

Al was sitting on the side of the bed several hours after the operation, was out of bed the next day, and on the fourth day he went home without any complications. Al was grateful to everyone involved in his care and let them know it.

I'm glad to say that Al never had a recurrence, and is alive and well today, continuing to make people happy and feel secure. You can bet his immune system and all other systems are working at max. He had an experience that caused stress, but his positive outlook guarded him against the negative effects of stress on his immune and other bodily systems.

Ben was another case entirely. His diagnosis was the same: cancer of the right colon. But there the similarity between the two men stopped.

When I told Ben about his cancer he reacted angrily, almost resenting me for telling him, even though I had tried to be as sensitive as possible in sharing the news. Ben wanted to see his x-rays. I showed them to him, even though surgeons themselves leave the interpretation of x-rays to the radiologist, who is the real expert in this field.

=========== Events That Cause Stress ===========

Events	Scale of impact
Death of spouse	100
Divorce	73
Marital separation	65
Jail term	63
Death of close family member	63
Personal injury or illness	53
Marriage	50
Fired at work	47
Marital reconciliation	45
Retirement	45
Change in health of family member	39
Pregnancy	39
Sexual difficulties	39
Gain of new family member	39
Business readjustment	39
Change in financial state	38
Death of close friend	37
Change to different line of work	36
Change in number of arguments with spouse	35
Mortgage over $10,000	31
Foreclosure of mortgage or loan	30
Change in responsibilities at work	29
Son or daughter leaving home	29
Trouble with in-laws	29
Outstanding personal achievement	28
Spouse begins or stops work	26
Begin or end school year	26
Change in living conditions	25
Revision of personal habits	24
Trouble with boss	23
Change in work hours or conditions	20
Change in residence	20
Change in schools	19
Change in recreation	19
Change in church activities	18
Change in social activities	18
Change in sleeping habits	16
Change in number of family get-togethers	15
Change in eating habits	15
Vacation	13
Christmas	12
Minor violations of the law	11

How many of these changes are associated with a serious illness? Check off changes that may have to be made when a serious illness comes, and add up the scale of impact points. Can you see why it is so important to have an inner defense against the negative impact of fear and of stress on your health?

After asking questions about his x-rays, Ben wanted a second opinion, which I welcomed.

He came back about two weeks later, and during our conference I strongly suggested that he transfer his care to the consultant, or to someone in whom he had complete confidence. There's nothing so difficult as treating someone who has no confidence in you. Ben's outlook was negative all the way, and I was uncomfortable with the atmosphere.

We had another conference, with his wife present, and went over the whole problem again, discussing all the probabilities and possibilities. Seldom do I place strong demands on a patient, but Ben seemed to require it. With his wife there I stressed the fact that he had a malignant tumor, which had to be removed in order for him to live.

Then I told him that I did not want to do the surgery; that I felt his lack of trust in me, and that it was important that he should trust whoever operated on him. That really upset him, because he did want me on the case. Ben just did not want the treatment.

But I was serious. I assured him his type of tumor was not rare, and that there were many surgeons in Seattle who could perform the surgery successfully. His wife was very supportive, and I think if it hadn't been for her he would never have submitted to the operation.

Finally the date was set, and I guaranteed I would do my utmost to make his course as smooth as possible. I visited each department of the hospital where I knew he would contact people—the admitting office, the lab, the floor nurses, and so on. I advised them of Ben's insecurity, and that he might give them a bad time. But I reminded them that he needed all our help to get over his malignancy.

When Ben was admitted, it went just as I'd thought. He was impossible everywhere he went. But the hospital personnel were wonderful and treated him as if he owned the place. They took a lot of abuse with no retaliation.

The worst scene of all came with the prepping of his bowel with the laxatives and enemas. I had rehearsed with him what to expect, but it wasn't enough. Finally he refused any more enemas, even though the return was not "crystal clear." After consulting with the crew who prepped the bowel, I decided he wasn't properly prepared. I went to his room to tell him his surgery would have to be postponed for a day in order to do a better prep and have a safe field in which to operate. Ben tried to talk me into going ahead, but I said the situation was not ideal. This was a time when we wanted everything in the best order.

Ben was so angry I thought he would sign himself out of the hospital, but he didn't.

The next day he went through the same routine again, and finally his bowel system was crystal clear.

The surgery itself went well, but as expected, trouble started as soon as Ben began to come out of the anesthesia. He asked for pain medication at the first sign of discomfort. He pulled out a necessary naso-gastric tube. The battle was on.

The nurses in the recovery room are pros; they had been through this before. They gave him sufficient medication to dull him and then let him know in a kind but firm manner what he had to do and why. If he didn't want to do it for them, they would do it anyway.

So he cooperated—in a way. He didn't like the deep breathing routine because it hurt. He didn't like the tube in his nose. Whenever he saw me he had a list of questions and complaints. He saw no sense at all in blowing up balloons—until he developed his first complication, a small collapse of a portion of his lung which could have been avoided if he had done what he was told. The next day he was told he was going to get out of bed.

"No way!" Ben thought his stitches would break and he would pop open.

He refused to move his feet up and down while in bed and would not turn from side to side. So he developed a clot in the deep muscles of the calf of one leg. This meant he had to have his blood thinned, because such clots can at times be fatal. I had a very serious talk with him, and from then on he left the treatment to us. But his hospital stay, which should have been no more than five days, stretched into fifteen. In fact, Ben was fortunate to get out at all!

Just for fun, I worked up a little check-list comparing and contrasting the two men and scoring each on a scale of 0 to 4, with a 4 being the highest score. Later, I found out that Al was a believer. But I really hadn't needed to be told.

Dealing with the stress of cancer:

	Al	Ben
Attitude	4	0
Faith	4	0
Confidence	4	0
Cooperation	4	0
Ability to cope	4	0
Ability to make decisions	4	0
Complications	0	4
Sense of humor	4	1
Gratefulness	4	0
Fear	0	4
General outlook	4	0
Ease of treatment	4	0
Complaints	0	4
Demands	0	4

The Faith Factor ═══════════

Dr. Herbert Benson, Associate Professor of Medicine at the Harvard Medical School, has long focused his efforts on studying the impact of stress on health, and on how to deal with stress. His first book, *The Relaxation Response,* became a national best seller and has helped to focus the attention of the medical community on the link between our emotional state and our physical health. In a new book, *Beyond the Relaxation Response,* Dr. Benson features what he calls the faith factor. He states:

> I've come to understand that the effects of this simple technique [the moment of quiet Benson calls the Relaxation Response], *combined with a person's deepest personal beliefs,* can create other internal environments that can help the individual reach enhanced states of health and well-being.*

Dr. Benson strongly emphasizes the importance of having confidence in one's doctor. But he goes far beyond this in arguing the importance of personal faith. He suggests that in about 25 percent of our ailments surgery or specific medications are the critical factors in recovery. But he then adds, "that leaves a notable *75 percent of situations where our personal beliefs can play a major role in healing physical ills.*"*

Dr. Benson carefully guards against making pronouncements about the merits of any specific belief system. He simply points out that faith, the confidence a person has not only in the doctor but in a higher power, makes a major difference in healing physical ills.

Now, personally, I want to go much further than Dr. Benson. As a Christian I don't simply believe in mind

---

Beyond the Relaxation Response by Herbert Benson, M.D. (New York: Berkley Books, 1985) pp. 5, 82.

over matter: I believe in God. I am sure that anything which brings a person a sense of confidence will be helpful in his recovery. But I am even more sure that a personal relationship with Jesus not only brings us the benefit of inner peace, but also permits our living God to work actively in and through those physical systems which He Himself designed. The Christian's faith factor is the most powerful faith factor of all, because our faith is in our living Lord.

I appreciate Dr. Benson's willingness to speak out strongly on the role of religious faith in helping a person be and stay well. That's a courageous stand to take, for the medical community is not especially religious.

In my practice, however, I've tried to go beyond this to help my patients develop faith in a caring God, and thus develop a solid basis for their hope.

Gloria was an attractive, exuberant, successful model and businesswoman in her early thirties when I first met her as a patient. She was referred to me because of a mass in her left breast. She was frightened, but kept her feelings very well hidden. She had extensive cancer of the breast, with metastases to the bone in her skull.

That's bad, since a metastasis is a transmission of the disease from the original site to other areas of the body. In other words, the disease had spread. I had to tell her as tenderly as I could.

During her postoperative period when I would see her in the office for dressings, I began feeding Gloria with hope, in spite of the medical findings. Little by little I told her about a power outside ourselves, and then pinpointed the living Jesus and His personal concern for her.

She never gave any indication that she even heard me, and when she left my care to start her chemotherapy and radiation, I considered her one of my failures. I felt I just hadn't gotten through to her.

About two years later, I got a call from Gloria. She wanted to make an appointment when I had some time to spend with her. I imagined I was going to see someone with extensive cancer, and that she wanted my advice. The day arrived, and I had cleared some time for her.

I was back in my consultation room, and I heard her check in with the receptionist. She came straight back and appeared at my door. And this gorgeous, healthy looking young lady said, "Meet your sister in Jesus."

It struck me like a bolt of lightning. She added, "You thought I didn't hear you all those times you talked to me, but I heard every word."

Jesus had spoken to her through my spirit, and the rest was natural growth, the satisfying of a hungry spirit. And another recovery from a cancer that by rights should have been terminal had happened.

As a result of that encounter, Gloria has been instrumental in inaugurating and directing a support group in Seattle called Cancer Lifeline. Gloria is alive today, filled with hope and confidence in Jesus, and encouraging others along the same way.

Christian Hope ════════

When we use the word "hope" in casual conversation, it's a rather weak term. When someone says, "I hope I can make it," he is really expressing doubt, not confidence. But for us Christians, "hope" has a different, vital meaning.

My friend, Dr. Larry Richards, has this to say about hope in his *Expository Dictionary of Bible Words:*

> Most often where we find "hope" in the English versions, the Hebrew word is *miqweh, tiqwah* (from the common root *qawah*) or *yahal*. Each Hebrew word invites us to look ahead eagerly with confident expectation. Each also calls for patience, reminding us that the fulfillment of hope lies in the future.
>
> *Qawah* forms focus attention on what it is that awaits us. In the Book of Job, perhaps the oldest OT book, Job

expresses the sufferer's fears as tragedy shatters his sense of comfortable relationship with God. "If the only home I hope for is the grave," Job cries, ". . . where then is my hope? Who can see any hope for me?" (17:13, 15). As Job faces his fears of the future, he rejects the suggestion of Eliphaz: "Should not your piety be your confidence and your blameless ways your hope?" (4:6). Ultimately Job finds the solution of the psalmist: "Lord, what do I look for? My hope is in you" (Ps. 39:7).

The psalmist, living after the time of Moses, was familiar with God's commitment to his people expressed in the covenants. God has always shown himself faithful to his commitment. God's specific plan for the future might not be fully understood; nevertheless, many psalms express an overflowing confidence in God personally. How God will deliver, in this life or for the life beyond, was not completely clear to these OT believers. But surely God was himself the kind of person who could be trusted.

Yahal forms dominate the psalms and the later prophets. This word for hope focuses on our present experience as we look ahead. At times translated "wait," *yahal* invites us to link our present relationship with God to hope. In this relationship the OT suggests that (1) God is a deliverer, who will act in the future to save the one whose hope is in him, and (2) it is appropriate for us to wait confidently until God acts.

Because the believer knows God and trusts him, the psalmist can say, "I will always have hope" (Ps. 71:14). When we have hope, we have courage to face each new day, for "the Lord preserves the faithful. . . . [Therefore] be strong and take heart, all you who hope in the Lord" (Ps. 31:23–24).

In a most basic way, then, "hope" is a relational term. It is a great affirmation of trust in God, not because the believer knows what is ahead, but because God is known as wholly trustworthy. David writes in Psalm 119:49–50, "You have given me hope. My comfort in my suffering is this: Your promise preserves my life." Again and again the OT exhorts us to hope. "O Israel," comes the invitation, "put your hope in the Lord, for with the Lord is unfailing love, and with him is full redemption" (Ps. 130:7).*

The Christian's hope is rooted in one thing and one thing alone. We know God, and we know that He is committed to us. In Jesus God has spoken a word of promise to you and me, and we rely on that promise.

I am convinced that a Christian who has grown in his or her personal relationship with Jesus has, in Christ, a hope—a positive expectation that good things lie ahead—which in Benson's words "can play a major role in healing physical ills."

Gloria illustrates it.

Al, whom we met earlier, also illustrates the faith factor. The positive outlook provided by confidence in Jesus and in His love lifted both of them, and played a vital role in their recovery. Ben, on the other hand, did get well, but his recovery was retarded by his fearful, insecure outlook on life.

As Larry has written, hope *is* a relational term. When we trust in God we have confidence, and look ahead optimistically. This is not because we know what is ahead, but because we know God to be wholly trustworthy. We can put our hope in the Lord, for His love is unfailing, and because with Him is full redemption.

I've known Mary for many years. She was a popular coed at the University of Washington. She had everything going for her—plenty of money and talent, and she was the envy of her friends because she was going steady with a super athlete. The world was Mary's oyster, and nothing could get in her way. Mary had a good sense of humor, and was the center of attraction wherever she was.

Expository Dictionary of Bible Words by Lawrence O. Richards (Grand Rapids, MI: Zondervan Publishing House, 1985) pp. 343–45.

She married her athlete, and he became very successful in the business world. The family seemed off to a great start. But gradually the fast lane lost its glamor, and there was a void that couldn't be filled. Mary should have been happy, but she found herself becoming more and more frustrated, to the point of becoming despondent. As time went on, Mary progressed into a full blown manic-depressive, with more periods of depression than mania.

Mary thought about suicide on several occasions, and became an ongoing psychiatric patient. There seemed to her to be no good reason to live, because life had no purpose.

Then in her treatment she saw a Christian psychiatrist, who had a great influence on her life. In fact, her consultations with him turned her life around and she has never been the same since.

This isn't to say that Mary's troubles are over. She still has depressed states. But now Mary has hope. She can see beyond her infirmity, and has never lost sight of eventual victory. Has Mary had victory? Is she well? Well, I can tell you this. Without her belief in the ultimate victory she would not be here today. Mary really believes in and depends on the strength derived from a real and personal relationship with her Lord.

I mention Mary because I don't want you to think that faith and hope in your Creator is some sort of magic pill.

I have to confess here that television healing services somehow don't appeal to me. I think there's too much emotion, and not enough substance. In many instances such services have been cruel, because an innocent victim has quit much needed medical care to rely on "faith" alone.

I also believe much so-called faith healing offers a false hope that is worse than no hope at all. Believers who pray earnestly to the Lord yet are not healed are likely to feel particularly guilty. If only they had enough "faith," they think, they would be healed.

If Mary had been programmed for that sort of hope, she would be even more miserable today than before. You see, Mary still has her down times along with the up. But Mary's hope is in the Lord—not in complete healing. And this is an important distinction.

Think about it.

Mary's hope is in Jesus.

Even when Mary is down, she knows God hasn't abandoned her. Even when she feels depressed, and especially then, Mary draws strength from the knowledge that God loves her and is with her.

Could God cure Mary totally? Yes. But in many ways her walk of faith is a greater witness to His constant grace than any miraculous cure could be. I know that Mary continues to be a real inspiration—to me, and to everyone who knows her.

You see, when our hope is in God, we trust ourselves to Him completely for whatever He decides is best.

Our hope isn't in a cure. Our hope is in God. We confidently expect that what God has in store for us will be good, because we believe God is loving and trustworthy.

With this kind of hope in God we have a peace that no sickness can destroy. We never have to feel guilty about the progress of our recovery because we have placed ourselves in Jesus' hands and our future depends on Him, not on ourselves or on the strength of our faith.

Hope for Now, and Forever

Senator Jones—not his real name—was a leader in our community. He owned the local newspaper, and knew everybody's business, but he was a real loner. He never smiled, never made small talk, and always seemed deadly serious. We all called him Senator Jones because none of us could ever feel close enough to him to call him by his first name.

Senator Jones became president of the hospital board, and I spent many hours with him at board meetings. Often when he was absent, the board members would talk about him, concluding that he was icy cold and just didn't like people. Did he have any friends? Where did he find social fulfillment? No one seemed to know. After ten years I didn't feel that I knew him any better than at first, and neither did anyone else. He did his job, and did it well. Apart from that, no one knew what he did or who he did it with. I studied him and tried to figure out what was going on inside, but he covered himself too well.

One day he became ill, and it turned out to be a very serious problem. He was about fifty, at the peak of his career. But before long he was confined to the hospital for treatment. He had cancer of the throat.

I thought a lot about Senator Jones, and one morning I went into his room. After all, I'd spent many hours in committee meetings with him. I said, "Senator, I just want you to know that I am sorry, and I am going to pray for you. I know you realize that you're in a tight spot, and I am truly sorry and upset. If there is anything I can do, please let me know."

He looked at me with a deep scowl, didn't say a word, and showed absolutely no emotion. I left the room thinking I had invaded his privacy and really blown it.

The next morning I came to the hospital early. The switchboard operator paged me, and said that the Senator wanted to see me. I thought I was in for it. Technically, I had broken the rules of the hospital. He was another doctor's patient, and I had told him I was going to pray for him without first asking his permission. This was against the hospital's patient privacy rule.

I hurried up to his room, and found him sitting up in

bed with his familiar scowl. "Good morning, Senator," I said. "What can I do for you?"

Slowly, but deliberately, he answered. "No one ever talked to me like you did yesterday. Why did you do that? What do you want?"

I assured him, "Senator, I don't want anything except what is best for you. We are all going to face what you are going through, and I happen to believe in a living God, who cares about you. I want you to know that same God. None of us can make it on our own. We all need help."

There was a pause, and then, "Tell me about your God. I've never been big on God, but I am willing to listen."

I gave him the good news of the gospel, and stressed the fact that God loved him so much that Jesus was willing to die for him. He drank it in. I stayed for about an hour, then I asked if I could pray with him. He consented. I placed my hand on his forehead and said just a brief prayer. His response was, "Will you please come back tomorrow?"

I saw him each day for the next week. Then he went home, and I continued to see him there. By then he was calling me Paul, and I was calling him Harold. Little by little I saw a very tender and loving spirit emerge. The cold, icy, impersonal Senator Jones was just a coverup, a mask. We had a wonderful two weeks together. He accepted Jesus Christ as his Lord and Savior, and I witnessed a transformation of this man. One night at home he hemorrhaged from his cancer and died. But he died in hope—the hope of life after death.

Did Gloria have hope? Yes, she found hope in Jesus. Jesus restored her to health and gave her a vital ministry to others suffering as she had from cancer.

Did Mary have hope? Yes, she found hope in Jesus. Jesus is in the process of restoring her now, and Mary draws strength from Him as she suffers with still-recurring bouts of depression.

Did Harold have hope? Yes, he found hope in Jesus. When Harold died a few weeks later, that hope was not disappointed but was fulfilled.

This is the real nature of Christian hope. Our hope is not in what we expect God to do for us, but in God Himself. When we trust ourselves to Jesus, and release our tensions and our fears to Him, we find peace.

In the majority of cases that I treat, I find that this peace has a dramatic impact on recovery. *Releasing it all to Jesus is one of the most vital of my spiritual secrets. It is one of the most vital of all steps that a person can take to find recovery and the restoration of vibrant good health.*

Developing Your Hope

In this chapter I've tried to point out how medical researchers now acknowledge that stress and fear are the deadly enemies of good health. In fact, they actually block recovery by supressing the immune system and affecting our other bodily systems as well.

These same medical researchers suggest that a positive, optimistic outlook enhances the effectiveness of our body's natural defenses against sickness and disease. Remember, *"Every change in the mental and emotional state, conscious or unconscious, is accompanied by an appropriate change in the physiological state."* Confidence in one's doctor and a firm religious faith both contribute to the changes in our mental and emotional state that bring about a positive change in our physiological state.

The faith factor makes a real, measurable, medical difference in our ability to combat disease!

For the Christian the faith factor is even more powerful. Our faith is focused in the person of the living God, who we know is real and who has complete personal concern for us. Christian faith leads us to the place where we can release all our fears and tensions to Jesus Christ because our hope truly is in Him.

How do we develop that Christian kind of hope which is expressed in the release of everything to Jesus, and in resting in Him? Here are some of the things I try to teach my patients, linked with the Bible verses for meditation listed on the next page.

First, remember that you are important to God because of who you are, not for what you do. God has shaped human beings in His image, and every one of us—including you—is truly important to Him. God loves you and values you. He values you so much that He was willing to give His Son so you could have eternal life. Sickness often brings depression and doubts. But the faith factor reminds us that such feelings do not fit the facts. God's love for us is a constant thing, for God has given Himself to us in Christ. We have hope in Jesus because of God's love for us.

Second, recognize the wisdom as well as the love of God. You and I are limited by our finitude. We can't see the future, and cannot tell the outcome of any series of events. Only God has the wisdom to look ahead and the power to guarantee the future. It is perfectly all right to tell God what we want, and to pray for specific healing. At the same time we must realize that God is committed not to what we think is best, but what He knows is best. We can hope in Jesus because of God's wisdom and power.

Third, consciously and purposefully place yourself in God's hands. Give Him your sickness. Give Him your future. Give Him your financial needs. Give Him your family. Release all your worries and fears to Him, for God has promised to care for you. When depressions or fears recur, remember and reaffirm this act of surrender. You are not "giving up." You are giving yourself into the hands of the Great Physician, who is able to work in your body as well as in your soul and spirit, and who alone can restore health. Rest your hope fully in Him, and let Him bring you peace.

Fourth, don't forget the practice of what I've called Lone Time. You need to nourish your personal relationship with God: to fill your heart and mind with renewed trust in Him. You can find suggestions for practicing your own Lone Times in chapter 3.

In the context of a growing personal relationship with the Lord you can remember God's love, recall His wisdom, and respond by consciously trusting yourself to Him.

As you put your hope and your faith in Jesus Christ, you release all the God-given powers of your body and are on your way to recovery. You are on your way to being truly well.

=========== **Reminders of Love** ===========

Fear not, for I have redeemed you; I have called you by
name; you are mine (Isa. 43:1).

My unfailing love for you will not be shaken nor my
covenant of peace removed (Isa. 54:10).

God sends his love and his faithfulness (Ps. 57:3).

I will not take my love from him, nor will I ever betray my
faithfulness (Ps. 57:3).

For God so loved the world that he gave his one and only
Son, that whoever believes in him shall not perish but
have eternal life (John 3:16).

In all things God works for the good of those who love him,
who have been called according to his purpose
(Romans 8:28).

God has said, "Never will I leave you; never will I forsake
you" (Heb. 13:5).

He sent his one and only Son into the world that we might
live through him. This is love: not that we loved God, but
that he loved us and sent his Son as an atoning sacrifice
for our sins (1 John 4:9–10).

=========== **Foundations for Hope** ===========

I pray . . . that the eyes of your heart may be enlightened
in order that you may know the hope to which he has
called you, . . . and his incomparably great power for us
who believe (Eph. 1:18–19).

I will strengthen you and help you; I will uphold you with
my righteous right hand (Isa. 41:10).

God will meet all your needs according to his glorious
riches in Christ Jesus (Phil. 4:19).

I am the Lord, your God, who takes hold of your right hand
and says to you, Do not fear; I will help you (Isa. 41:13).

May the God of hope fill you with all joy and peace as you
trust in him, so that you may overflow with hope by the
power of the Holy Spirit (Rom. 15:13).

Let him who walks in the dark, who has no light, trust in the
name of the Lord and rely on his God (Isa. 50:10).

"For I know the plans I have for you," declares the Lord,
"plans to prosper you and not to harm you, plans to give
you hope and a future" (Jer. 29:11).

Part II

Spiritual Secrets
of Staying Well

6

Lifestyle

Choices

In the first section of this book we looked at the spiritual secrets that affect recovery from serious illness. Now we're ready to look together at something that may be even more important—the secrets of staying well.

Researchers tell us that over half the problems for which adults consult a doctor involve only 25 percent of the population! *I want to see you in the 75 percent that has less than half the medical problems!*

After forty years of medical practice and after carefully studying the medical literature, I've become convinced that good health is directly linked to our lifestyle. While some of these lifestyle choices are obvious, others are rather subtle.

Joe was a professional man and very successful. At the age of forty he entered politics, and again success

followed him. The only problem was, the more successful Joe became the more he drank.

It sneaked up on him, really, and in spite of warnings
Joe was sure he could control his drinking.

Then one morning his picture appeared on the front
page of the paper. Cited for driving while intoxicated,
he had been involved in an accident in which a child was
seriously injured.

Joe tried to go on the wagon, and he did have some
success. But he soon fell back into his old daily drinking
habit.

I followed Joe through the years. After a time he
began doing strange things and forgetting important
appointments. During conversations it became clear
that he was having difficulty tracking and was unable to
think things through logically. I referred Joe to a very
sharp neurologist, who examined him and then called
me. His diagnosis was chronic alcoholic brain damage,
with no possible chance of reversal.

Joe had destroyed the thinking part of his brain with
alcohol.

Joe lost his political office, his standing in the community, and little by little, his resistance to infection. Finally he succumbed to an overwhelming infection—a
real tragedy for such a bright and promising man.

Ted was a successful go-getter too. He was a friendly
man with a ready smile and a lovely home and family.
And he took care of his health. He watched his diet, and
he worked out regularly at the same gym where I go.

But then Ted began to change. He lost some of his
friendliness, and began to miss his gym workouts because of minor sicknesses.

What had happened was that Ted, despite a loving
and attractive wife, had begun an affair with one of the
girls at his office. This led to a series of sexual misadventures. But it also led to a growing sense of guilt, and

an inner stress that upset the balance of his immune system. Ted's illness and unhappiness were a direct result of his wrong moral choices.

Finally Ted faced his guilt and found forgiveness. He returned to his wife and family with a renewed commitment. Gradually, the stress was relieved, and Ted rebuilt not only his home but also his glowing good health.

Tom was a young attorney who came to my office and told me he had vomited some blood that morning. All symptoms pointed to a bleeding ulcer which was not too bad at the moment. He had lost some blood, but his total blood count had not fallen significantly.

I made arrangements for Tom to go into the hospital where we could treat him and monitor his blood loss. But he didn't go into the hospital. Instead he went to his office. And then he went on a call to deliver some papers. He totally ignored medical advice because he felt okay and had no pain.

While walking along the street, Tom became faint, collapsed, and was rushed to the hospital. He stabilized in intensive care after receiving several units of blood. Tom was then taken to surgery, and I tied off a very active squirting artery. Then I completed the ulcer operation.

When I got to the hospital I had told Tom, "You are going to be okay." He'd been afraid I would chew him out and embarrass him in front of the staff. "But you didn't even mention that I hadn't followed your advice."

Later Tom laughingly called himself a "slow learner." But he did learn. When he was well and ready to go back to work, we sat down and talked about his lifestyle. Why did he have an ulcer in the first place? It soon became clear that Tom was a workaholic. His life and personal relationships were far out of balance. I laid out steps he could take and we talked of how to incorporate them in his daily routine. Tom has done this faithfully. Today he's a better husband, a better father, a better friend, and a better Christian. And his ulcer has never returned.

These three individuals illustrate what I mean by lifestyle choices. Joe made the choice to abuse his body with alcohol. That choice led directly to his ruin and death. Ted made wrong moral choices. The stress created by his guilt also led to illnesses and a loss of well-being. When Ted found forgiveness and committed himself to the right moral path, he found his health returning. Tom made more subtle choices. His choice to focus totally on his work and to set aside other values and relationships led to an ulcer, while a reordering of his priorities led him back to health.

These are the kinds of things I want to think about with you in this chapter, and in the chapters that follow. What lifestyle choices are you making? And how do these choices affect your health?

I'll be blunt in these chapters. I'll give you the advice I've given my own patients, and I'll share some of the medical evidence that supports my advice.

I can't and won't try to make your choices for you. But as a physician and as a Christian friend, I want to help you see clearly the implications of the choices you may be making now, and the choices you can make in the future.

I was amused when I read a quote from Harold Burson's talk to the Tenth Symposium on Medical Education, held at the New York Academy of Medicine. Burson said:

A physician friend of mine once gave me his prescription for making patients happy. The first thing you have to do is guarantee them immortality; you have to guarantee them that they will be here forever. And after you do that, you must guarantee them full sexual vigor during the entire course of their lives. Finally, you have to make all this possible at little or no cost, and with a minimum inconvenience or change in lifestyle.

Well, I can't always make my patients happy since I cannot guarantee immortality or lifelong sexual vigor, but I do want them to be well. I want you to be well.

And, believe me, for many of us wellness will come only with a significant change in lifestyle!

So let's look at the lifestyle choices that affect our health, and through it all I want to reassure you that God did create you and me to be well. He supplied us with the physical systems needed to keep us well. And God's Word supplies us with guidance that will help us keep those systems functioning as He intended.

Substance Abuse

Tobacco: I recently went to a medical seminar attended by some five hundred doctors. It was a fascinating experience. Just ten years ago, that room would have been hazy with smoke. This time not one of the five hundred doctors was smoking!

Today we have positive evidence of the harmful effects of tobacco products. We know the link between smoking and lung cancer, heart disease, and emphysema. We know the cancers caused in young people by smokeless tobacco. If you wonder how strong that evidence is, all you have to do is consider the fact that 90 percent of the doctors who smoked have quit!

I've mentioned some of the effects of tobacco in earlier chapters. I won't repeat them here. I'll only say that smoking is a clear and present danger to you—and to others in your family who may breathe in your second-hand smoke! If you want to be well, and if you smoke, quit.

Alcohol: Alcohol is the most dangerous drug in America today. It is a depressant that has serious consequences, and it is not advisable for any possible medical purpose.

Jean was about fifty when she came to see me for a chronic illness. She hadn't been feeling well for about a year, and for three months had been getting rapidly worse.

Her symptoms consisted of nausea, loss of appetite, weakness, and a fullness in her upper abdomen. In the past three weeks her skin had begun to take on a yellowish cast. The nausea got worse, and her abdomen became larger.

On examination it was clear that her liver was greatly enlarged; and that she had fluid on her abdomen. The blood studies, along with the physical symptoms, revealed that she was in acute liver failure from cirrhosis of the liver due to use of alcohol.

Jean had confessed to drinking wine, but she hadn't thought of alcohol as a possible culprit in her present problem. How was I going to tell her?

I sat down by her bed and told her we had all the information. We knew now just what her problem was. I had to tell her that she had liver failure, and to explain the probable terminal outcome. And I had to tell her that her drinking was the cause.

"Why, that's impossible!" she said indignantly. "I drank only wine."

Well, whether you get it in wine, beer, or liquor, alcohol is alcohol. And alcohol has an affinity for two of your most sensitive bodily systems: the nervous system and the liver.

Even a small amount of alcohol in the bloodstream goes immediately to the brain. There it impairs judgment and prolongs reaction time. Thousands of people, many of them completely innocent, are killed or maimed because others who have been drinking choose to drive. More work hours are lost, and more domestic problems are caused by alcohol abuse than any other reason.

Liver cells are very sensitive to alcohol, too. The first change seen under a microscope is swelling. The cells become distorted, and then begin to die. As this happens, scar tissue and fat are deposited, and new liver cells are formed. The process of new cell formation is so active that the liver becomes enlarged, sometimes up to ten times! At the same time, the scar tissue blocks the blood flow through the liver, and the condition known as cirrhosis develops. The abdomen may fill with fluid, and gallons may be tapped off due to back pressure. Back pressure can extend to the veins of the esophagus. These in turn can rupture and cause acute bleeding and vomiting. This type of bleeding is difficult to treat and control. Many a night I've stayed up with someone who was bleeding from a ruptured vein of the esophagus.

These patients are poor risks for surgery and demand intensive care. Even then, the outlook is bleak, and recurrences are high.

The liver is hard to insult. But once it is done, the person will never be the same again. When a doctor taps, as I have, literally gallons of fluid which have collected in the abdomen from back pressure due to liver failure, there's no question of being convinced just how toxic alcohol is.

And to compound all that, alcohol has a dramatic way of neutralizing vitamins, and recently has been shown to alter the effectiveness of the lymphocytes of our immune system.

Street Drugs: We are a society that is becoming increasingly health conscious. Yet at the same time we have an increase in consumption of tobacco, alcohol, and drugs. Unfortunately, the users appear to be becoming younger and younger, and they seem to be using more and more of these products.

The frightening thing to me is that the drugs used are highly addictive and cause permanent damage to the psyche. What used to be considered a "safe" drug, cocaine, is recognized today as being extremely dangerous.

Cocaine acts much like an amphetamine in the initial stages. It arouses the user and makes him feel euphoric. It reduces fatigue, and generally makes a person feel on top of the world. But the effects of cocaine are short-lived. The user needs to take frequent doses to satisfy his hungers, and he tends to use increasingly larger doses.

We now understand what happens when people use this drug. Cocaine neutralizes a normal chemical in the brain called dopamine. Prolonged use of cocaine results in shorter and shorter highs, and a deterioration of the body. Euphoria turns into depression and confusion, leading to paranoia and dementia. If depressed sufficiently, the lack of dopamine will cause a person to go into shock and die.

Cocaine is both physically and psychologically addictive, and continued use of this drug can lead to permanent brain damage.

Over-the-Counter Drugs: Over-the-counter drugs, or non-prescription drugs, are now plentiful. Most of them are not harmful if taken as directed. The one which gives us concern is the diet tablet which contains phenyl-propanolamine (PPA). PPA is used in most diet pills and stimulates the metabolism. It also activates the nervous system and can lead to psychological disturbances. In addition, it increases the pulse rate as well as the blood pressure. It is not a good medicine to take for weight loss.

The other drug that you can buy over the counter is caffeine. Caffeine is a stimulant and increases the pulse rate as well as the blood pressure. It also stimulates the central nervous system, which leads to alertness followed by depression. Caffeine users, either by tablets or coffee, tend to gradually increase their dosage. The eventual result is frayed nerves, or harm to the heart, blood pressure, and psyche.

Put simply, the lifestyle which promotes health will also eliminate substances which depress or attack the immune and other systems God intended to keep us healthy.

The use of tobacco, alcohol, or *any* street drugs unquestionably distresses the systems that are responsible for good health. We can choose to be well by refusing to make such substances a part of our lives.

Morality Abuse

When Ted turned to sexual misadventures he made a wrong moral choice. And that moral choice had an impact on his health.

The problem with sexual immorality isn't simply with the host of STDs (sexually transmitted diseases) you can contract. The problem with sexual immorality, and with other sinful moral choices, is that such choices affect the inner *you,* and that in turn affects your health.

Ted's sense of guilt affected his ability to fight off infection. He became fatigued. He lost his sense of joy in his work and his ability to concentrate. In Ted's case he also showed allergic symptoms he'd never had before. The stress of his moral choices had upset his immune and other bodily systems.

As a doctor, I know that our emotional and mental state has a dramatic impact on our bodies. As a Christian, I know that our moral choices—whether or not we are believers—have a powerful effect on our emotional and mental state! Why is this?

The Bible tells us that God created a moral universe, and populated it with people who have a moral sense. This does not mean that any person is sinless. We all fail. But it does mean that everyone is born with an awareness of right and wrong.

In the Book of Romans, Paul points out that even pagans living without the benefit of God's law "do by nature things required by the law" (2:14). Every society operates with a moral standard that includes rules for proper and improper sexual behavior. It's the same in other areas to which God's law speaks. The standards of pagan societies may not be identical to biblical standards. But the point is that standards do exist.

In the same passage, Paul argues that "they show that the requirements of the law are written on their hearts, their consciences also bearing witness, and their thoughts now accusing, now even defending them" (2:15).

When a person's conscience accuses him or her of doing wrong, pagans try to deal with it by accusing themselves ["I am guilty," "I am a failure," "I am no good," and so forth] or by excusing themselves ["It wasn't my fault," "He is to blame," "You'd have done the same if you were me"]. Each of these approaches to dealing with guilt is futile. The first depresses the mental and emotional state and drags down a person's health. The second also stresses the mental and emotional state, leading to bitterness and anger, which also drags down a person's health.

The more a person violates his conscience and tries to deal with that violation by accusing or excusing, the greater the adverse effect on his or her health.

It's no wonder that Ted, and the hundreds of others like him whom I've seen, become sick. Their sinful moral choices have violated their consciences and thrown them into a helpless cycle of sin and self-recrimination.

The Christian has two answers to this dilemma. Each is illustrated in a story told by Dr. William Wilson of Duke University:

> Rose was a thirty-two-year-old mother of two who had been terribly neglected and traumatized as a child by her wealthy parents. Both parents spent too much of their time in social activities and, as is often the case, drank excessively. Her father could easily be classified as an alcoholic, since he was subject to drunken rages during which he would abuse his wife and children.

To rid themselves of the burden of their children they left them in the care of "nannies" and other servants. It was only logical that very early in life Rose felt rejected.

After she finished high school her parents refused her request to go to college. She was sent to a finishing school in Europe to learn how to "catch a right husband."

Unable to rebel against her parents, she went to Europe and began to drink heavily and was sexually promiscuous. After she came home she made her debut, and very soon thereafter did what was expected. She caught the right husband.

He was right, because he was energetic and creative and made enough money to keep her in the manner to which she was accustomed. In only a few months she became pregnant, and in due time had her first child. At this point Rose realized that she was drinking too much, but could not stop. After her second child was born she realized that she was an alcoholic, but her husband was much too busy to respond to her pleas for help. How could he know that she was telling him the truth? He was never at home.

Rose made a second futile try to get her husband to help her, but again he ignored her. She then decided that, since she seemed to be following in her father's footsteps, she might as well do what he had done a few years before. She would commit suicide.

Fortunately, she had been befriended by a Christian neighbor who recognized her distress. Before she had a chance to carry out her plans, this friend had arranged for her to see me. When I examined her I was fully aware of the severity of her depression, but she denied any suicidal intent. So I treated her with antidepressant medications. She promptly used these to attempt suicide. I admitted her to the hospital.

Shortly before her discharge I was discussing her past history with her when she revealed how horribly guilty she felt about her escapades during her finishing school years. As I listened, I realized that I had not dealt with her guilt, so I said to her, "But you are forgiven."

Startled, she looked at me in amazement and said, "I am? Who forgives me?"

I responded, "God does, and I do."

Suddenly she began to weep and said, "Oh, thank you, God! Thank you, Dr. Wilson."

During the next hour I told her of God's love for her, and how through His Son she had received forgiveness. At the end of the session she accepted Christ as her Savior. She was discharged a few days later.

After her discharge from the hospital her friend invited her to a Bible study, and to a church known for its warm fellowship. She accepted both invitations eagerly. Rose also continued in psychotherapy with me for the next year, during which time we dealt with the unhappiness of her childhood. Her subsequent life has been filled with happiness. She has remained sober and has served the Lord well.

In her prayer for salvation, Rose surrendered her life to Christ to do with what he willed. Such a surrender is a radical step for my patients, but it is usually necessary if the patient is to be healed of such problems as alcoholism, drug addiction, sexual perversions, or severe personality and characterological problems. Surrender of one's will allows God to guide and direct complete healing of these persons.*

This was the path Ted took too. First came acceptance of Christ's forgiveness for the sinful choices he had made. Then came a surrender to Jesus, and the decision to live a new kind of life.

The solution to the wrong moral choices that have created stress and that will, sooner or later, destroy health, is found in first accepting God's forgiveness, and then making fresh choices to do what is right.

Today our society is too tolerant of moral deviations. We form committees to support the "rights" of those who insist that their moral perversion be recognized as simply an "alternative lifestyle." We watch TV soap operas that

---

*From an unpublished speech, used by permission of Dr. William Wilson.

feature adultery and sexual promiscuity, and suggest that such actions are the norm for everyone. Our government gives price support to growers of the tobacco which slowly kills other citizens. And, all too often, drunk drivers, instead of going to jail, are simply released to drive drunk and perhaps to kill again. Too many in the business world argue that their "sharp" practices are what everyone does, and that they have to do the same thing to succeed. And some of our districts re-elect to public office those whose private immoralities have been revealed.

It's not surprising that some think they can adopt a lax moral standard for themselves.

But they can't.

This remains a moral universe, and God has built into human beings a moral sense and sensibility. The person who chooses to sin will find his choices rob him not only of the blessings of God, but also of peace and health! Isaiah said it long ago in words that describe the emotional and mental state of those who choose to act against what they know is right and to sin.

> But the wicked are like the tossing sea,
>> which cannot rest,
>> whose waves cast up mire and mud.
> "There is no peace," says my God,
>> "for the wicked" (Isa. 57:20–21).

Choosing Your Lifestyle

I can sympathize with folks like Rose, whose circumstances bring almost unbearable pressures. And even for men like Ted, who face daily temptations. And there is nothing like the pain of sitting beside a woman whose drinking or smoking has brought her life to a premature end.

But while I feel sympathy, I can't excuse them.

And I don't excuse you.

God has still given you and me the power of choice. We are responsible moral beings.

And what good news this is! It means that your future and my future aren't determined by our past. Someone like Rose can still find forgiveness, and win release from the grip of her habits. A Ted can face his sin, accept forgiveness, and make a renewed commitment to his wife. A person who has smoked can choose to quit, and a person with an alcohol habit can turn his back on the past.

Something the apostle Paul wrote to the Corinthians is exciting to me. It tells me that the things which frustrate and tempt me as well as my patients are things that are common to us all. We're all subject to the stresses of life, and all must make choices.

But that same verse tells me that in God I have the resources that I need to win over my temptations. I'm given the resources I need to make the right choices in my life. My personal relationship with God, found first in Jesus and nurtured by time alone with Him, will free me from the things that have bound me. With the strength God gives me I can make the choices that bring new balance to my lifestyle, and will move me toward the constant enjoyment of vital good health.

If you ever feel weak, or doubt your ability to choose the right path, hold on to this promise from God's Word: "No temptation has seized you except what is common to man. And God is faithful; he will not let you be tempted beyond what you can bear. But when you are tempted, he will also provide a way out so that you can stand up under it" (1 Cor. 10:13).

What a wonderful promise to grasp. So why not reexamine your lifestyle, reexamine the choices you have been making, and appropriate God's promise to help you choose His good way? Then choose. And be well!

7

Diet and Exercise

The most common physical problem in North America is obesity. As a people, we're just too fat.

And, as a people, we just don't exercise enough. These two problems go hand in hand, and believe me, they're serious. Anyone who is eager to live a truly healthy, whole life needs to take a careful look at his or her diet and exercise program.

One diet doctor, a specialist in weight loss (a person called a bariatric internist) shocks people who come to him by telling them in the first interview, "You have more chance of recovery from cancer than of recovering from obesity."

He does it to shock his patients into realizing that weight loss demands commitment. But the remark isn't particularly encouraging.

Actually, I won't tell you that weight loss is next to

impossible. And I won't give you any fad diets, or rigorous exercise programs to follow. What I will say is that you *can*, by making a few basic lifestyle choices, lose your excess weight and build up your body's strength and stamina. It will take some personal discipline. But you can make several simple diet and exercise decisions that will enable you to be, and to stay, well.

What's Fat?

As a general rule, obesity is defined as a body weight 20 percent over the midpoint of the weight range given in standard height/weight tables. Unless you're heavily muscled, this is a pretty accurate definition.

Just recently there's been some debate over those height/weight tables. The tables that insurance companies use changed from 1959 to 1983. And in 1985 the National Institute of Aging noted that desirable weight can and should change with age. Laying down a little fat as a person grows older can be a good thing. But again, only a little—and certainly not more than 20 percent of the midpoint of that recommended weight. And, by that definition, one in every four Americans is fat!

But why is being fat a problem? While some of my patients have been unhappy because their fat makes them feel unattractive and depressed, I'm more concerned about what fat does to the bodily systems that God designed to maintain our health. Simply put, being fat is dangerous!

What are the dangers? Well, for one thing, heart attacks are more than twice as frequent in overweight people. Strokes are six times more frequent. Fat persons also show an elevation of norepinephrine and of an enzyme known as renin, which causes high blood pressure and hypertension. Then there is a condition called hypercholesterolemia, which is an increased amount of fat in the blood. Fatter persons have an increased incidence of high blood sugar, or diabetes. When you put these

What is my desirable weight?

	Metropolitan Life Insurance Co. 1959 table (In pounds for ages 25-59)		1983 table		National Institute of Aging 1985 recommendations for both sexes (In pounds by age in years)				
Height	Men	Women	Men	Women	Height / 20-29	30-39	40-49	50-59	60-69
4'10"		91-119		100-131	4'10" 84-111	92-119	99-127	107-135	115-142
4'11"		93-125		101-134	4'11" 87-115	95-123	103-131	111-139	119-147
5'		96-125		103-137	5' 90-119	98-127	106-135	114-143	123-152
5'1"	107-136	99-128	123-145	105-140	5'1" 93-123	101-131	110-140	118-148	127-157
5'2"	110-139	102-131	125-148	108-144	5'2" 96-127	105-136	113-144	122-153	131-163
5'3"	113-143	105-135	127-151	111-148	5'3" 99-131	108-140	117-149	126-158	135-168
5'4"	116-147	108-139	129-155	114-152	5'4" 102-135	112-145	121-154	130-163	140-173
5'5"	119-151	111-143	131-159	117-156	5'5" 106-140	115-149	125-159	134-168	144-179
5'6"	123-156	115-147	133-163	120-160	5'6" 109-144	119-154	129-164	138-174	148-184
5'7"	127-161	119-151	135-167	123-164	5'7" 112-148	122-159	133-169	143-179	153-190
5'8"	131-165	123-155	137-171	126-167	5'8" 116-153	126-163	137-174	147-184	158-196
5'9"	135-174	131-165	139-175	129-170	5'9" 119-157	130-168	141-179	151-190	162-201
5'10"	139-174	135-170	141-179	132-173	5'10" 122-162	134-173	145-184	156-195	167-207
5'11"	143-179		144-183	135-176	5'11" 126-167	137-178	149-190	160-201	172-213
6'	147-184		147-187		6' 129-171	141-183	153-195	165-207	177-219
6'1"	151-189		150-192		6'1" 133-176	145-188	157-200	169-213	182-225
6'2"	155-194		153-197		6'2" 137-181	149-194	162-206	174-219	187-232
6'3"	159-199		157-202		6'3" 141-186	153-199	166-212	179-225	192-238
6'4"					6'4" 144-191	157-205	171-218	184-231	197-244

together, you've got coronary heart disease, with a high risk of heart attack. No wonder the National Institute of Health emphasizes that a body weight of 20 percent or more above that midpoint "constitutes an established health hazard," and has called obesity a "killer disease"!

Actually, none of our bodily systems works to its optimum in the face of obesity.

But the fad diets that many fat persons turn to are often as bad as being fat! In this book I've stressed the importance of the immune system. The functioning of that system depends on a normal, healthy blood count. There are white blood cells in the blood which are the protectors of our health. One type of white blood cells takes care of acute infections. The other, called lymphocytes, takes care of the more complicated problems, including cancer. As I've mentioned before, we all probably have cancer cells in our body all the time. But cancer begins to spread and take over only when conditions are right.

One of those conditions is a deficiency of certain amino acids, the building blocks for proteins. When the amino acids decrease, our antibodies become abnormally low, and then we are susceptible to infection or cancer. When the amino acids are deficient, the immune system suffers. The specialized T and B type lymphocytes are decreased, suppressing our first line of defense. With immunity depressed, there's a downward spiral that's terribly difficult to reverse. For example, antibiotics will not work in an immune-deficient person.

According to studies, deficiencies of vitamins A, E, B-6, and some minerals are associated with reducing the effectiveness of our immune systems. But the effectiveness of the immune system is also reduced by an excess intake of fat, and by excess zinc, iron, or vitamin E.

It seems like a real dilemma. Eating can lead to problems. And not eating well can be just as troublesome. I've seen people go from one fad diet to another, and in the process get into big trouble because *those diets do not provide good nutrition.*

As a matter of fact, I'm not in favor of dieting to lose weight. I just don't believe that counting calories, or fad diets, will help you deal with your weight problem.

But at the same time, I have to say that if you're a person who is at least 25 percent overweight, you're a sitting duck for problems. You have no choice but to get the weight off, as soon as possible. The key to losing weight is to eat a balanced diet with the right amount of proteins, carbohydrates, and fats to keep you and all your systems at optimum health.

A little later in this chapter I'm going to show you *how* to lose and keep weight off. In fact, I'll show you how to avoid that terrible yo-yo effect most overweight people have experienced, of losing pounds and then suddenly gaining them back almost overnight. I'll show you how to enjoy eating, and save hundreds of dollars, too.

But first, let me comment on a few common but false beliefs associated with diet and nutrition.

Dietary Fallacies

1. *"Fat in childhood, fat for life."* This notion is based on something that we do know about obesity. If a child is fat, he or she has a four-to-one chance of being fat in adulthood. If an adolescent is fat, that chance increases to twenty-eight to one. But the old theory that a fat baby develops extra fat cells and retains them into adulthood just isn't true. An adult can develop extra fat cells just as easily as a baby.

It is true that there seems to be a heavy genetic factor in overweight people. If a parent, especially a mother, is overweight, there's a good chance that one of the children will inherit whatever it is that predisposes to obesity. But the fact of the matter is that for 95 percent of us, being fat is a choice that's linked to our lifestyle! Except in the most unusual cases, you can control your weight by diet and exercise.

2. *"Carbohydrates are bad for you."* Carbohydrates have had bad press, but not for any good reason. Take a baked potato for example. That carbohydrate-rich potato is an excellent source of bulk, and of vitamins B and C. It doesn't even have too many calories (until we smother it with butter and sour cream and bacon bits).

Usually the notion that carbohydrates are bad is linked with the idea that proteins are good. Many diets have proposed that the way to lose weight and keep it off is to eliminate the carbohydrates and fill up on the proteins. But there are problems with this approach.

It's true that a high-protein diet tends to suppress the appetite. But it is also true that excess protein is processed by the liver, reduced to amino acids, and that the excess amino acids are then sent to the kidneys which excrete them as urea. Your body doesn't store any of the excess protein. In fact, those excess proteins only add stress to your liver and kidneys which have to process them chemically before they can be removed from your body. So why overwork these organs by stoking up on hundreds of excess protein calories?

3. *"'Natural' foods and food supplements are important."* There are problems with processed foods these days. The prepared foods we buy in our supermarkets tend to have far too much salt, and far too little fiber. But the notion, encouraged by so-called health food stores, that much of the nutritive value in food has been destroyed or removed in processing, and that supplements are needed, is so much hype! So is the idea that the replacement foods and supplements you need must be "natural."

In the first place, all vitamins and minerals are "natural." Whether a vitamin is produced in a laboratory or by a plant or animal, its chemical structure is exactly the same. And minerals, like calcium, magnesium, sodium, potassium, manganese, and zinc are exactly the same whatever their source. *The fact is that in a well-rounded diet the vitamins and the minerals we need are plentiful.*

Then why buy expensive dietary supplements in those health food stores? I don't know any good reason—unless you like to spend money unnecessarily.

I do, though, remember one interesting surgery. Carl was in serious trouble with an impacted intestine. Nothing would pass through. It was clear that we had to operate.

Carl had a stretch of intestine that was packed with some material that was literally as hard as cement, and I had to cut out that section.

After the operation I talked with Carl to try to find out what had caused his problem. He was adamant that he hadn't been eating anything that might cause problems. In fact, he said, he was careful with his diet, and ate only naturally grown vegetables. And he also used a variety of dietary supplements found at his local health food store.

That was it. Oh, yes, the supplements contained all the vitamins and minerals advertised. But these vitamins and minerals came in capsules *which were largely filler.* Carl had taken so many capsules that the sandlike filler had built up in his bowel, hardened, and without the operation could have killed him.

4. *"We need more vitamins and minerals than normal eating can provide."* This notion is extremely popular with some people. The idea that we need massive doses of vitamin C to fight off cancer and the common cold has even achieved the status of folklore.

The virtues of vitamin C have been argued by Dr. Linus Pauling, who suggests 7 or 8 *grams* of vitamin C a day. This is 160 times the amount recommended as the daily requirement by the National Academy of Sciences!

What happens to all that extra vitamin C? It passes through your system. First, the body does not store excess vitamin C. Second, the lining of the intestine is very selective. It absorbs only what is needed to keep the immune system in a healthy state, and to provide the minute quantities needed by other cells. What is not absorbed is carried to the kidneys, and excreted as urine.

It's the same with most of those other vitamins that we take in megadoses. They simply pass through.

As someone has remarked, Americans must have the most expensive urine in the world!

Supplemental minerals aren't needed by healthy individuals either. Fluoride is adequate in most water supplies. Zinc and iron and the rest of the minerals we need are well supplied in a varied diet. However, a menopausal woman *is* prone to osteoporosis (softening of the bone). We do recommend a calcium supplement to avoid this complication. But don't rush out to a health food store. Just drop in to your corner drug store and buy some Tums. It's your cheapest form of calcium, and just as effective as the most expensive form you could buy.

5. *"Processed sugar is bad, and should be replaced by 'natural' sweeteners like honey."* Sugar is often maligned as providing only "empty calories." It's true that sugar provides no vitamins or minerals. And yes, sugar is a carbohydrate and the excess is deposited as fat. It's also well documented that sugar is a cause of dental caries. While this is a good reason to brush your teeth after meals, it's not a reason to give up sugar entirely!

Sugar is not a poison. It's actually a fuel, a source of the energy your body uses to burn fat, and a source of the glycogen your body stores in muscles for reserve strength. And, it takes a lot of sugar to make you fat. One teaspoonful of sugar equals eighteen calories. A teaspoon of butter contains forty-five calories!

If sugar is all that bad, why do all doctors use sugar solution intravenously in hospitals as a base vehicle to supply nutrition?

The fact of the matter is that sugar can be used, sparingly, to make food appetizing. It's excess sugar, like an excess of most other things, that causes us problems.

And as for the notion that sugar is "artificial" and "bad" while honey is "natural" and "good," there is no significant difference nutritionally between honey and sugar! Both provide "empty" but nonetheless essential fuel calories.

6. *"All cholesterol is bad."* Everyone these days seems to have heard that cholesterol is linked with heart disease. Fatty cholesterol deposits can build up in blood

vessels and are a major cause of heart attacks. A blood test will reveal if the total cholesterol level is under 180, which is considered normal. And the test will measure the type of cholesterol present. Remember, cholesterol isn't *bad*. We need cholesterol to have healthy cell walls in all tissues, and we need it for the formation of the antibodies in our immune system.

The thing is that both *too much* cholesterol, and the *wrong kind* of cholesterol, can create health problems. We classify cholesterol by the type of lipoprotein it contains. There is high density (HDL), low density (LDL) and very low density (VLDL) cholesterol. It turns out that the lower the density lipoprotein the cholesterol is made of, the worse it is for your blood vessels. It is the lower density cholesterol that sludges, and causes a waxy substance to stick to the walls of the small arteries, especially of the heart and kidneys. HDL cholesterol does not do this.

Now, the kind of cholesterol in our body depends on the lipoproteins we feed our body. So where does the low density protein in our systems come from? Primarily from red meats, egg yokes, and other animal fat like butter. Fish, especially salmon and shell fish, is very rich in HDL and actually lowers the total blood cholesterol, plus reducing VLDL and LDL.

If our protein sources emphasize fish and chicken, and even vegetable proteins, we won't have high levels of the wrong types of cholesterol.

7. *"All fat on your body is the same."* We've learned a lot about fat metabolism. For instance, the type of fat you eat is the type of fat you deposit. If you eat vegetable fat, you deposit vegetable fat. And if you eat animal fat, you deposit animal fat. This has been proven by chemical analysis of fat deposits.

A Swedish study shows that men and women deposit fat in different places. Women deposit excess fat primarily on hips, thighs, and buttocks. And this is a more stable fat than that deposited in other places, which means it's the last to go! I've seen many women exercising, dieting, and losing pounds—only to be disappointed that their hips have not gone down. Yes, they lost fat. But not in the right places.

Men on the other hand have a predisposition to deposit fat in their abdomens, both inside and out.

But before a woman envies a man, consider this. That hip fat may come off more slowly. But it's abdominal fat that is most closely linked with heart trouble and other diseases associated with obesity.

8. "*Additives and preservatives are bad for you.*" No one argues the fact that fresh produce, right out of the garden, is a first, best choice. In the same way, we'd all like freshly baked bread. But those of us who live in the city, or in climates where fresh vegetables won't grow all year around, don't have that option. We eat bread and other foods with preservatives. And we eat vegetables that have been washed with sulfites to keep them from turning brown.

One popular view is that such preservatives and additives are poisoning us. The notion is that the chemicals are carcinogenic (cause cancer) and have all sorts of harmful effects.

The fact is, the chemicals are by far the lesser of two evils. Sulfites won't hurt you unless you have an allergy to the chemical. Preservatives won't hurt you either. The Food and Drug Administration constantly runs tests on the various additives for toxic effects. And if we did not use such chemicals the food we now enjoy would spoil during transport from the farm to the consumer. The bread we eat would be moldy. And the mold of spoilage *has* been shown to be carcinogenic!

Looked at this way, believe me, the standard chemicals that keep our food from spoiling are a blessing. We need the protection they provide.

I could go on and list scores of other notions about diet that have become part of popular folklore. We could look at many other fallacies that have led Americans to spend approximately seven billion dollars each year on totally unnecessary and sometimes harmful food supplements. We could analyze those diets with the exotic names, and the ones associated with some doctor or celebrity, and show why each all-new, $14.95 diet program is actually nutritionally extreme.

But what I want to do in this chapter is give you a simple prescription for a way of eating that will promote and maintain vigorous good health. Essentially, what I plan to tell you is to eat, and to enjoy eating—but in moderation.

Eat and Enjoy

I don't believe in extreme diets.

And I don't believe in those strict diets that tell you to carefully count out your 900 calories as you starve daily.

There are two reasons. First, unless you have a lot of support and someone to whom you are accountable daily, you won't follow through on that diet or count those calories. Second, what every person needs to develop is an *eating lifestyle*. What will make and keep you healthy is a way of viewing and enjoying food that will give you the nutrients you need to keep you healthy coupled with the exercise pattern I'll suggest later, to keep your weight under control.

It is true that God has provided in the basic food groups all we need for vibrant good health. You can eat well, enjoy your food, and be perfectly healthy. And you'll save all that money some pay for health foods and unnecessary vitamin supplements.

On pages 128–131 I've laid out a simplified approach

to eating that, if followed, will help you lose weight and give you lifetime weight control. It will provide that good nutrition so important to good health. And you'll be able to enjoy eating without constant worry about calories. Before you look at it, let me explain some of the principles on which my Lifetime Eating Plan is based.

The rules for my Lifetime Eating Plan are extremely simple. *Eat a low fat, moderate carbohydrate, moderate protein diet, with fresh fruits and vegetables.*

That's it.

If you eat a low fat, moderate carbohydrate, moderate protein diet with fresh fruits and vegetables, you'll maintain good health.

Now, I can expand on and explain that prescription. But we never need to change it.

What do I mean by expanding and explaining? Well, it's best not to get all your protein from red meat. Vegetable proteins and the proteins in fish and chicken are better for you. So I encourage you to get a moderate amount of proteins from these sources.

Fresh produce is best, with frozen next, and canned vegetables last. Freezing causes the loss of very few nutrients, including vitamins. But canning causes a considerable vitamin loss.

In that low-fat, moderate carbohydrate, and moderate protein diet you'll also want to eat a variety of foods. Choose whatever you like from various categories of food: fruit and vegetables, meat or meat substitutes, low-fat dairy products, breads and cereal. Those four categories of nutritious foods will provide all the fat, protein, carbohydrates, vitamins, and minerals you need. Make sure you get a variety of these foods, and you'll be okay.

You'll notice in the diet plan on these pages I don't get specific and tell you which foods from each category you should eat. Why should I? I don't know your likes and dislikes. Why should I tell you to eat broccoli if you hate broccoli? You can just as easily have a substitute you like.

I also don't tell you to count calories. Just check your scales. Or take a look in your mirror. If you don't like what you see, eat smaller portions. Keep the portions under control, and you'll lose weight—*and* have all the nutrients you need for good health.

Let me give you one word of encouragement. Crash diets and fad plans are often designed to give a quick, spectacular initial weight loss. When you follow my prescription, and adopt the weight loss program I suggest, you probably won't lose a lot of pounds right away. Why? Because on a lower protein, lower carbohydrate (and thus fewer calorie!) diet a person tends to retain salt and fluid. As a result, the scales may not change much at first. *But you will be losing fat.* Change in the scales will come later.

In fact, if you're trying to lose weight, I suggest that you *do not weigh yourself* daily. I wouldn't even mind if you weighed yourself only every month or so. That way you won't be discouraged even when your weight begins to yo-yo. By staying with the program your weight will get down, and stay down, and your health risks will also be reduced.

Your high blood pressure and high blood sugar will return to normal. Your cholesterol level will return to normal. And then you'll be in smooth water, safe from the dangers that lurk ahead for the obese.

And remember, that's what each of us is really looking for. Not a diet that will take our weight down dramatically, only to be followed by another sudden weight gain. We're looking for a pattern of eating that will help us control our weight and provide all the nutrients we need for glowing good health.

The great advantage to the weight loss program I recommend here is that you will lose weight gradually, restoring your systems to healthy balance while developing an approach to eating that will enable you to enjoy food while you remain healthy—for life.

A Lifetime Eating Plan

I've told you some of the principles. Here are the specifics. You'll need to get about 20 percent of your calories from fat, about 30 percent from protein, and another 50 percent should be from carbohydrate, primarily complex carbohydrates.

The typical working man needs about 2500 to 3000 calories daily to maintain weight. About 1200 calories makes for good, steady weight loss. So my *Diet Worksheet* on page 130 is designed to give you 1200 calories *in the desired proportion.* If you're not on a diet, simply double the amounts, *but keep the same proportions.* Adjust the amounts for your own size and activity, *but keep the proportions the same!*

Here are the food groups you can choose from, with approximate portions. There are many foods not listed here, but these are the basics in our American diet.

Dairy Products

Skim milk   1 cup
Lowfat milk   1 cup
Plain yogurt $^1/_2$ cup

Vegetables

$^1/_2$ cup or 1 medium-sized vegetable constitutes a serving. Eat only one serving each day of those marked *. Eat as much as you want of the others.

Artichokes*
Asparagus
Beans (green,yellow)

Beets*
Bean Sprouts
Broccoli
Brussels sprouts
Cabbage
Carrots
Cauliflower
Celery
Cucumbers
Eggplant
Mushrooms
Onions*
Parsley
Peppers
Peas*
Pumpkin*

Radishes
Squash (any kind)*
Tomatoes
Zucchini

Protein Sources

Eat primarily fish, chicken and turkey. Limit cheese, eggs, and red meat. Serving size is 1 oz.
Cheese
Chicken
Cottage cheese ($1/2$ cup)
Eggs
Fish
Red meat
Shellfish
Turkey

Fruits

Servings are $1/2$ cup, or 1 medium fruit, except where indicated.
Apple
Unsweetened applesauce
Apricots (2)
Banana ($1/2$)
Berries
Cherries
Dates (2)
Grapefruit ($1/2$)
Melons
Orange

Peach
Pear
Pineapple
Plums (2)
Tangerine

Complex Carbohydrates

Except where indicated a serving is 1 slice or $1/2$ cup

Breads
Baked beans
Cold or hot unsweetened cereal
Corn
Crackers (6 squares)
Lima Beans
Pancake (1 small)
Rice
White or Sweet Potato

Fats

Use plant fats rather than animal fats. Serving is 1 teaspoon except where indicated.

Margarine
Salad Dressing
Mayonnaise
Nuts (6 to 10 whole nuts)
Oils (cooking)
Seeds

Choose your foods from these lists and keep the proportion established in the Diet Worksheet, even when you increase the amount you eat. This will provide a balanced, healthy diet that will help you be and stay well.

=== **1200-Calorie-a-Day Diet Worksheet** ===

To lose weight, eat the number of units of each of the foods listed in this chapter each day. Plan your diet around the foods you enjoy. Just *check off* each unit as you consume it to keep track of what you eat. The size of a unit is defined in the comments above the list where the food is found (see pages 128–129). This worksheet page may be duplicated and used to chart your own weight loss diet each day.

Dairy Products
☐ ☐

Vegetables
☐ ☐ ☐

Fruit
☐ ☐ ☐

Complex Carbohydrates
☐ ☐ ☐ ☐

Fats
☐ ☐ ☐

Proteins
☐ ☐ ☐ ☐

Other
   ☐ You may season with one tablespoon of simple carbohydrates (sugar, honey, and so forth) each day.
   ☐ Enjoy all the unflavored gelatin that you want.
   ☐ Add a tablespoon of unsweetened taste-fresheners such as horseradish or mustard.
   ☐ Include one cup of a clear soup as a snack if you wish.

Exercise ═══════════

Physical exercise is as important to good health as the food you eat.

By physical exercise I mean *serious* exercise that extends the major muscle groups and raises your pulse rate to flush out all the smaller arteries, including the coronaries. A fast flowing stream will not as easily deposit cholesterol plaque in the walls of the arteries.

For me this means regular workouts under a professional trainer at a downtown Seattle gym.

Even though I'm past seventy, these aren't easy workouts. Harry, who is the best physical fitness expert I've ever seen, watches me and his other charges carefully, changing our routines to work every muscle group. One of the routines he designed is called the "Iron Man Ten." He has had us alternate running a flight of stairs with running a lap of the gym. One "lap" of the stairs was a down-and-up routine of 44 steps. Harry started us off with a set of laps, and worked us up to ten sets. At that level we lapped 55 flights of stairs and 55 laps of the gym. Like I said, that's not easy!

Harry always watches us closely and checks our pulse rate regularly. For those in good condition Harry allows the pulse to increase to 150 beats per minute, and to hold it there for two minutes or so, and then gradually lower the pulse rate from 150 to 120. When in good condition a pulse should drop to under 100 after two minutes. (Please do not try to raise your pulse to 150 until you are in top condition!)

Now, I know that not everyone has access to a gym and a trainer like Harry. So I'm not going to suggest you have to join a health club and work out daily. I just want you to know that I am so convinced of the importance of serious exercise that, years ago, when I was a busy physician and surgeon, I found the time to begin and to maintain a serious exercise program.

I still maintain that program today.

And I'm still busy. I'm busy in my capacity as a member of the King County Medical Society's Grievance Committee, and as its public relations officer. I'm busy in my role as a medical consultant to various government agencies.

But I'm not too busy to exercise daily.

I'm delighted to see so many people exercising today, and recognizing the need to keep in shape. Believe me, being in shape makes a world of difference in how a person feels. It certainly improves resistance to infection. And it decreases complications from surgery, should that occasion arise.

I mentioned above that I realize not everyone can find a trainer like Harry, or have access to an outstanding gym. So, what should a person do—particularly when sedentary exercise, like golf, can't meet the criteria set up for serious exercise? I've mentioned those criteria. Let me state them again. Serious exercise *extends major muscle groups* and *raises and maintains a higher pulse rate.*

A couple of activities that meet these criteria are active tennis and vigorous swimming.

But what if you can't play tennis, and don't have access to a swimming pool? Well, there is one exercise that is available to everyone. It doesn't require expensive equipment. It doesn't call for driving to a special location. There are no fees or tuitions to pay. That exercise is *serious walking.*

What is serious walking? It is walking briskly with long strides, swinging your arms and breathing deeply. You can start out walking vigorously for as little as five minutes (about a half mile) a day. This should be gradually extended until you're walking for forty-five minutes to an hour a day. At that level, warm up by walking less vigorously for five or ten minutes, walk *seriously* for twenty to thirty minutes, and then walk less vigorously again to cool down.

Where will you find the time to walk? That's up to you. Perhaps a walk will fit in your morning schedule. Or perhaps in your lunch hour. Believe me, you'd be better off skipping lunch and walking than not walking at all. Evening is a good time for a serious walk, and has the added benefit of getting the tensions out of your body, relaxing you, and preparing you for sleep. Again, *when* you exercise is up to you.

If you want to truly be well, a good exercise program is as important as a balanced, nutritious diet. God *has* provided, in the world He created, all the foods we need to maintain the function of our bodily systems. And He has so designed our bodies that, if we eat properly and exercise, we can expect a full and a healthy lifetime. If you treat the body God has given you wisely, taking care what you eat and how you exercise, I truly believe that you can expect a better quality of life. You can expect to be well.

8

Spiritual Renewal

John was a very sick ten-year-old when his father rushed him to my office. His appendix had burst and peritonitis had set in.

John's dad, Ken, was a supersalesman, extremely successful. Ken and his wife were both caught up living in the fast lane. But when John got sick, it really affected his dad.

I had to sit down and tell a distraught Ken, "I want you to realize exactly where we are. Your boy is very sick. He has an overwhelming infection, and I can't tell you yet whether he'll make it. But I can assure you we'll do all we can." And I went on to explain the treatment.

For the first day or so Ken was just beside himself. So I made him an unusual offer. "I get down here to the hospital about 6:30 in the morning," I told Ken. "I'll see John first of all. Then you and I can go to breakfast together, and I'll tell you just what's happening. You leave me phone numbers of where you'll be all day, and I'll call you if anything happens."

Little by little, John overcame that infection. About the tenth day, I was able to tell Ken at breakfast, "John is going to make it."

Later, when young John was out of the hospital and at home, Ken and his wife visited me. Ken said, "Boy, have I learned. I've learned what life is all about."

Ken and his wife *had* learned. There was a complete change in their lifestyle. They became a very close family, doing things together. They began to go to church. Ken was still a supersalesman, but he was no longer dominated by a competitive drive to succeed and make money. His priorities and those of his wife changed significantly as their outlook on life shifted from the materialistic to the spiritual.

Later the family moved to Connecticut. For years we heard from them at least twice a year, and when we visited the east Ken took time off from work to show us around.

Oh, yes. There was one other significant fact. Ken had had an ulcer. After John's illness, and after the family priorities changed, Ken's ulcer disappeared.

Ken had been healed spiritually—and physical healing followed naturally.

I've seen it so many times. I saw it in Larry, a driver on our Metro bus system. "Mean" was the best word to describe Larry. He *was* mean: opinionated, impossible to get along with, and dominating toward his wife, Rhoda. As you might expect, Larry didn't have many friends.

Then he was stricken with MS (multiple sclerosis). In most cases MS proceeds slowly, in a series of declines and remissions that may stretch out for many years. In Larry's case the disease was rapid and progressive. He was gone within two years.

But in that time, Larry changed. He told me, "Dr. Paul, I used to think I had to work hard to make a lot of money. But there's no such thing as security in this world." Suddenly aware of spiritual realities, Larry literally became a loving man. Even in his sickness he was always on the lookout for some small thing he could do for others. By the time Larry died, he had friends all over the place.

And then there's Clyde. Clyde was a tough taxi driver—a man who drove his cab at night and knew the seamy side of life. He literally saw life in the raw, transporting prostitutes, gamblers, you name it.

Clyde suffered a ruptured appendix with complications. In the course of treatment he became a close friend of mine. In fact, when he worked the day shift, Clyde would pick up some little old lady who'd give him a doctor's office address. Clyde would ask, "Who are you going there to see?" When his customer told him, Clyde would say, "You don't want to go there. I'll take you to see a *good* doctor." And then he'd bring his customer to my office.

I wasn't looking for new patients, but there was no use telling that to Clyde!

Then Clyde became seriously ill. And he, too, underwent the kind of change I've described in Ken and Larry. From a tough, cynical, and materialistic man Clyde became a sensitive person attuned to eternal values. Clyde, in fact, became a very spiritual person.

In each of these cases a tragic sickness was the catalyst God used to give someone rushing to destruction an opportunity to reevaluate the meaning of life. In each case, physical sickness led to spiritual renewal. In each case, old values were tested, found wanting, and replaced with new values that gave an entirely new perspective on life.

In Ken's case, spiritual renewal followed his son's illness, not his own. And that spiritual renewal, with the change of perspective it always brings, led to the healing of Ken's serious ulcer problem.

I've seen it again and again. Sometimes a life-threatening or life-ending sickness will bring spiritual renewal. *When the typical person experiences spiritual renewal, physical healing generally follows.*

Why a Spiritual Renewal? ═══════════════

To me, several things characterize a spiritual person. First, of course, there is a deep personal relationship with God through Jesus Christ. Along with that very personal relationship, I've noted two significant traits. The spiritual person is not a materialist. His or her idea of the meaning of life isn't bound up in money and possessions. And the spiritual person is a caring individual. Loving relationships with other persons are important to him or her. On the other hand, the materialist tends to *use* rather than *value* persons.

Seeing the impact of the materialistic and the spiritual perspectives on health has fascinated me for years.

I am convinced that the materialistic perspective only adds stress and distress to our lives. When stress becomes *dis*tress, our health *will be* affected.

I can't help thinking here of a person I've known for years. He was so anxious to get ahead he would do almost anything to achieve his goal. He's now wealthy, but lonely. He's not fun to be around, and never has been. He wonders why he has no friends, but does not realize it is the fruit of his own greed. Why should he? He's been like this all his life. He has used many people, and then deserted them. He has taken, but not given. Yes, he's wealthy. But his life is empty, and he is not only miserable but is, in the deepest sense, unwell.

What are some of the characteristics of the materialist that create inner distress? Here are a few that I've noted over the years.

Materialistic people tend
to measure "success" in terms of money
to expect satisfaction from things
to be excessively competitive
to think they can progress at someone else's expense
to be unhappy with what they presently have
to devote most of their time and effort to work
to have little time to spend with family or others
to be emotionally isolated: to have no one with whom
    to share feelings and needs
to find their achievements unsatisfying
to value what others can do for them, but not value
    others for who they are
to be anxious
to be lonely
to be self-centered.

Believe me, tendencies like these are a prescription for unhappiness—a stress that becomes distress leads to a loss of health.

The Bible speaks often of the foolishness of materialism. As my metro bus driver friend found when MS struck, Jesus was right when He taught that "a man's life does not consist in the abundance of his possessions" (Luke 12:15).

It is fascinating to find in the Bible so many insights into the psychological and spiritual implications of materialism.

For instance, Jesus noted that a focus on material things serves to create anxiety. After all, earthly treasures are subject to theft and destruction. Nothing about them is truly secure. In contrast, a spiritual focus relieves anxiety. Instead of desiring more possessions, or even worrying about necessities, the spiritual person remembers that God is a heavenly Father who knows our needs. We trust God to supply us daily because we know that we are truly important to Him (Matt. 6:19–34).

Paul warns that people who want to get rich fall into one of the devil's traps. He notes that a love of money is a root of all kinds of evil. When the desire to be rich replaces the desire to please God, persons will choose evil means to reach their ends. But evil always creates guilt, and guilt is one of the most destructive forces of all (1 Tim. 6:6–10).

Some of our most fascinating insights come from the Old Testament. The prophet Habakkuk was upset because he saw the wicked prospering at the expense of the more godly. How could God permit such injustice? When Habakkuk appealed to God, God explained a number of principles of judgment that operate as natural consequences in this moral universe of His. The first principle analyzes the impact of the warped desires on the wicked. The prophet is told:

> Indeed [this] wine betrays him;
>   he is arrogant and never at rest.
> Because he is greedy as the grave
>   and like death is never satisfied (Hab. 2:5).

What is Habakkuk saying? Simply that the desires of the wicked can never be satisfied. Like a furnace which becomes hotter as more fuel is added, each fresh achievement merely feeds the desires of the greedy. No matter how much he gets, he will hunger desperately for more.

What a horrible state! The more you get, the less satisfied you are. As you reach one goal, your hunger becomes greater, not less. And the emptiness within is simply enlarged.

The Psalms also make an important contribution. Asaph, one of the psalmists, found himself jealous of the wicked. The wicked seemed to live at such ease, without any of the troubles Asaph himself was experiencing.

Finally God gave him a fresh perspective, and he realized that ease was really "slippery ground." The seemingly easy life of the wicked leads directly to pride and arrogance. They never awaken to their need for a relationship with God, and as a result when troubles do come or death approaches they are emotionally "destroyed, completely swept away by terrors" (Ps. 73:19).

These biblical descriptions are accurate, penetrating analyses of what happens in the spirit and soul of a person who adopts a materialistic perspective on life.

He or she becomes anxious.

He or she is tempted to do wrong, which creates guilt and intensifies anxiety.

He or she becomes more and more dissatisfied, and life seems increasingly empty.

He or she becomes proud and arrogant, but completely unable to handle the tragedies that come into every life.

And every one of these traits has been shown to depress our immune system!

Every one of these traits has adverse effects on our other bodily systems. Every one of these traits tends to create stress, and to transform that stress into distress. Every one of these traits is linked with sickness, not with health!

That's why, speaking strictly as a medical doctor, I am convinced that people need to experience a spiritual renewal. A person who truly wants to be and to stay healthy simply must get rid of a destructive, materialistic perspective on life, and replace it with a healthy spiritual perspective.

Spiritual Renewal

I pointed out earlier that spiritual renewal begins with a personal relationship with Jesus. It doesn't end there. We need to continue deepening that relationship.

In the process we need to let Jesus reshape our values and priorities.

It might help here to profile the traits that I've noted in persons who have experienced what I call spiritual renewal. Such persons, whose perspectives are shaped by spiritual rather than materialistic values, tend

to live within their means
to have a circle of close friends
to give time and effort to family relationships
to empathize with other people
to have friends with whom to talk about personal
    problems and needs
to be givers, reaching out to help others
to truly enjoy the good things of life
to develop Christian friendships
to belong to a small study or prayer group
to take time for relaxation and vacations
to have a thankful attitude

I hardly need to say that this lifestyle tends to reduce rather than increase stress, not that anyone can totally *avoid* stress. But spiritual values and perspectives equip us to deal with stress in a healthy, positive way.

The person with a spiritual perspective is far better equipped to cope with stress than the person with only a materialistic outlook on life.

The foundations for this spiritual outlook on life are laid in clear biblical teaching.

The first line of teaching is designed to release us from our anxiety. It's summed up in a familiar passage, but one we need to look at again, and sense the force of what Jesus is saying:

> You cannot serve both God and Money. Therefore I tell you, do not worry about your life, what you will eat or drink; or about your body, what you will wear. Is not life more important than food, and the body more important than clothes? Look at the birds of the air; they do not sow or reap or store away in barns, and yet your

heavenly Father feeds them. Are you not much more valuable than they? Who of you by worrying can add a single hour to his life?

And why do you worry about clothes? See how the lilies of the field grow. They do not labor or spin. Yet I tell you that not even Solomon in all his splendor was dressed like one of these. If that is how God clothes the grass of the field, which is here today and tomorrow is thrown into the fire, will he not much more clothe you, O you of little faith? So do not worry, saying, "What shall we eat?" or "What shall we drink?" or "What shall we wear?" For the pagans run after all these things and your heavenly Father knows that you need them. But seek first his kingdom and his righteousness, and all these things will be given to you as well. Therefore do not worry about tomorrow, for tomorrow will worry about itself. Each day has enough trouble of its own (Matt. 6:24–34).

There are several things to notice in this passage. *First,* our viewpoint will be oriented either to God or to the material world. As Jesus said, no one can serve both God and money. A choice has to be made.

Second, choosing God brings us into a Father/child relationship with Him. In that relationship God commits Himself to meet our material needs, because we are so greatly valued by Him. The spiritual perspective helps us understand how truly significant we are as individuals. God loves us deeply, and in love commits Himself to care for us.

Third, there is a vital inner impact of the discovery that we are truly important to God, and that He is fully committed to us as our Father. We are released from anxiety. The pagans "run after" food and drink and clothing—life's necessities—because they live in an impersonal universe. They must depend on themselves alone, and so are filled with fears and uncertainty. Believers are released from this kind of anxious worry about tomorrow and freed to enjoy the blessings of today as they put God and His kingdom first.

I've known many Christians who've never made the basic choice of God over money, of the spiritual over the material. They may know Christ as Savior, but they have not gone on to orient their lives to the Lord. These believers are caught in the trap of materialism and still show the anxieties and fears which place stress on our immune and other bodily systems. Spiritual renewal, that reorienting of our life and values to God rather than to material things, is something many Christians need to experience.

The second line of teaching is designed to refocus our relationships with others. This line of teaching is summed up by Jesus, who gave His disciples a new commandment: "Love one another. As I have loved you, so you must love one another" (John 13:34).

Recent studies by Drs. Jane and John Dixon of Yale University have shown the importance of social connections as a health factor. In a nine-year study following up some seven thousand residents of Alameda County in California, those with the least extensive social and community ties had a higher death rate than those with the most extensive ties. Physical exams also showed that the group with the least social connections and community ties had a high incidence of hypertension (high blood pressure), infections, heart disease, arthritis, colitis, and migraines.

Do you realize the significance? Here are secular studies confirming well-known Bible truths. Jesus advised community. Where people get together and have community, loving bonds with others, there is a healing element.

And when people get together to praise and pray, there is a power that cannot be measured.

It can be medically demonstrated that our bodily systems do not work as well when a person tries to go it alone. We were *meant* to be social, we were meant to have warm and close relationships with others. Only with such relationships—vertical with God, and horizontal with others—can we have wholeness of body, soul, and spirit.

But let's go back to Jesus' command. When He called for love (community), He gave us an additional definition.

We are to learn to love others—to be caring, sensitive to others' needs, willing to serve them—as Jesus has loved us.

What Happened to Hank?

Hank was a father who loved his son. But his was a domineering love. He stressed discipline and correction, and all the time he felt he was doing his duty and being a good parent.

I've taken care of Hank and his family for years. He's a successful merchant with a driving personality. He makes all the decisions, and is obviously in charge. I've watched Hank's son, Dean, grow up. I watched Hank prime Dean to take over his business. There's no question that Hank loves his son. He just wants Dean to be his clone, to do and think just as he does. At the same time Hank was totally blind to the fact that he was emotionally crippling his son.

Dean became increasingly quiet and introverted, to the point where he had no confidence and was losing the respect of workers around the store. Dean also began developing neuroses in the form of anxiety attacks, headaches, dizzy spells, insomnia, loss of appetite, and depression. Dean's marriage deteriorated, and finally broke up. You may have guessed it: He began drinking. His life was miserable.

Finally Hank came to me in desperation for advice. I made an appointment for the next day, when we could have a long period of time together. We went over the entire history of what had happened, and then pinpointed the problem.

The problem was Hank.

At first Hank resented it. But little by little he began to see the picture. Fortunately his wife also understood the problem, but she had never been able to talk to her husband. Gradually, Hank rebuilt his relationship with Dean. And Dean has responded beautifully.

He's quit drinking. He's remarried, and seems to be secure in his new marriage. And Dean is now in charge of the store, and doing very well.

Hank is having a difficult time staying out of the driver's seat, but he is definitely doing better.

I see the son regularly, and he's helped by talking with someone who knows the situation and can help him cope. Dean is still on medication, but much less than before. His anxieties are disappearing and he sleeps much better.

It's not a perfect situation yet. But Hank is working on his problem.

That problem? A crushing kind of love, that can actually cause the illness of a loved one.

That's why Jesus had to go on to define the love that makes for community. It's not just caring for people that gives God's new direction to live. It's this: "*As I have loved you*, so you must love one another" (John 13:34).

How excitingly these two lines of teaching mesh! A person who is released from materialism by deepening faith in God is redirected to a concern for people rather than for things.

Redirection follows release. Suddenly we realize that we are not intended to use people to gain things, but instead are intended to use things to serve people.

With this realization our whole system of values and priorities changes. We are launched on a way of life that brings health not only to us, but to others as well.

Jimmy's Story ━━━━━━

Jimmy was a little old man who lived with his wife. But the rigors of modern living caught up with both of them. They were a proud couple and wanted to make it by themselves. But, little by little, they found that their savings were not going to take care of them. Some luxuries to which they had become accustomed had to go, medical care being one of them. So they dropped their medical insurance.

You guessed it. Soon after their coverage was dropped, Jimmy developed symptoms of fatigue, shortness of breath, pitting edema (swelling) of the ankles, and a pounding pulse.

The shortness of breath became so bad he could no longer do ordinary chores around the house, and he was forced to seek medical help. Jimmy was in congestive heart failure, but with a few tests and medication he began to improve.

He did need medical attention at regular intervals, and that taxed his finances. Jimmy didn't say anything. But it came to the attention of the doctor that he was paying five dollars a month on his bill—a pretty good sign that he was struggling. A little investigation revealed he was going without essentials to pay his medical bill.

The doctor bill was immediately marked "paid in full" and returned to him.

Jimmy was in the office the next day to point out the error. When he was told the doctor had forgiven his debt, he broke down and wept. Not only was that bill "paid in full," but the medicine he needed was provided, and the family finances were continually enriched by "unknown friends" who wished to remain anonymous.

This was the best medicine that couple could have had, because it meant someone cared.

Who got the most good out of the transaction? You can bet the doctor and his staff went home feeling fulfilled and needed. A church became involved and ministered in a way that protected Jimmy but did not smother or make the couple feel obligated. Everyone involved sensed the power of love, not just to meet physical needs, but to bring a sense of fulfillment, joy, and self-worth.

That's what is so therapeutic about Jesus' kind of love. In loving others as He has loved us, we not only serve them but we fulfill ourselves. In the fulfillment that comes from serving we find joy and peace—a peace that brings spirit, soul, and body into harmonious relationship with each other and with God.

I'd never claim that the Bible is a medical text. But the Bible *is* a book that reveals how to live with God and others. It's a book on how to live with ourselves. It's a book that shows us what the Creator intended our life on earth to be like.

Holy Harmony

When we live according to God's plan a beautiful harmony is created between spirit, soul, and body.

And when that harmony exists, one of the many benefits we experience is good health.

I've given you a couple lists of my own, drawn from my observations of the characteristics of materialistic and of spiritual persons. The Bible has the same kind of lists. One matched pair of lists comes from the book of Galatians. One list describes those who live out of harmony with God, dominated by that dimension of the human nature which can't see beyond the material universe of touch, feel and grasp. The other list describes a person in touch with God's Spirit, and committed to spiritual priorities.

Just look down these two lists. Compare them. And imagine yourself to be characterized first by the one set of traits, and then by the other.

The materialistic individual	*The spiritual individual*
sexually immoral	loving
impure	joyful
debauched	peaceful
hateful and antagonistic	patient
discordant	kind

The materialistic individual	*The spiritual individual*
jealous and envious	good
given to fits of rage	faithful
selfishly ambitious	gentle
given to drunkenness and the like (Gal. 5:19–21)	self-controlled (Gal. 5:22–23)

Now read them over, and as you do, ask yourself: Which way of life brings stress? Which brings tensions? Which brings into a person's life those terrible strains which destroy the balance of one's immune and other physical systems?

No, the Bible isn't a medical textbook. *But the Bible does describe a way of life that is healthy.* And it warns against a way of life which is destructive to health.

What a tremendous blessing it is to be a *Christian* doctor! What a privilege over the decades to do more than just prescribe medicines and do surgery.

As a Christian doctor I truly believe I've been able to share with my patients spiritual secrets that offer them not only recovery but a lifetime of vigorous good health.

And how glad I am that I've had this opportunity to share my final spiritual secret with you: Choose, and live by, God's priorities.

As you develop and live by Christian values, I truly believe that you will *be well.*

9

Uniquely You

I suppose it's something of a cliché to say, "You're special."

But it's true. Each of the patients I've treated in over forty years of medical practice has not only been special, but he or she has also been unique.

I'm often caught up in the wonder of it. Of all creation, there is only one you, only one me. Only you have your fingerprints. Only you have your eye color. No other person's body functions exactly as yours does. No one reacts exactly the same way to illnesses, or even to medicine as you do.

That's why as a doctor I have to tune in to the individuals I treat: Even people with "identical" problems are so different that what works for one may have no effect on the other. Perhaps that's why the practice of medicine, for all our technological advances, is still an art.

That uniqueness is compelling evidence to me of how very special you are to God. He has made you to be *you:* No one quite like you has ever existed in the past or will exist in the future.

Those "differences" between you and others are special, loving gifts of a God who has such concern for the individuals that the very hairs of our heads are numbered and accounted for (Matt. 10:30). With the psalmist we can each say:

> For you created my inmost being;
>   you knit me together in my mother's womb.
> I praise you because I am fearfully and wonderfully
>   made;
>   your works are wonderful,
>   I know that full well.
> My frame was not hidden from you
>   when I was made in the secret place.
> When I was woven together in the depths of the earth,
>   your eyes saw my unformed body.
> All the days ordained for me
>   were written in your book
>   before one of them came to be (Ps. 139:13–16).

Meet Eddie

Eddie was one of God's special people. He was born to a wealthy and successful businessman. As a young boy Eddie developed diabetes, which kept him from normal activities. His father became overprotective, and Eddie soon resented this "loving" protection. He saw his dad as a deterrent to independent growth, and an obvious rift developed between father and son.

Eddie was a free spirit. He tended to ignore his diabetes. But his diabetes was the juvenile type, which tends to do the most severe damage to other structures, especially blood vessels and kidneys. Hypertension and heart disease are commonly associated with this type of diabetes. The skin flushes easily, and the typical rosy cheek look is often present.

Eddie had them all, but lived a full life in spite of his problems. He married a beautiful woman and had two daughters. They were an ideal family, and really got the most out of life. Eddie always wanted to be independent, but his father was a continuing threat to that independence. His resentment became so strong that his wife at one point asked me to talk to Eddie's dad—not a very comfortable role. I tried, but didn't make much of an impression.

But Eddie kept on making the best of his problems. He lived within his limitations, and accomplished more than most of his healthier counterparts. He viewed his disease with a certain amount of disdain, and didn't allow the symptoms to deter him from a normal life.

Eddie and his wife became people of strong faith, and I had the privilege of being with them in a small Bible study group. His insights were profound and personal. Perhaps that spiritual gift of insight was developed because of his tenuous health. But at any rate, Eddie learned how to be very ill, and yet to be well.

In his thirties, Eddie began having serious problems. He was treated at the university for what became progressive and more serious complications, including heart and kidney failure. Before long he slipped into an irreversible state from which he never recovered.

The last time I talked with Eddie, he was happy, not complaining, and very optimistic. He was looking forward to the return of Jesus, and in the next life to a far better body.

Was Eddie Well? ══════════

Eddie was an outstanding and creative person in spite of his affliction. Eddie was special and, even though his health was handicapped, in the deepest sense Eddie was truly well.

I've seen many people like Eddie over the years. I've treated people who have lost limbs. People who have lost their sight. People who have lived with chronic illness.

I couldn't promise them new limbs or new eyes in this life. I couldn't offer Eddie new kidneys or a new heart. But what I could do was to help each person find health—wholeness and fulfillment—within his limitations.

Let me say that again.

My goal as a healer has been to help each person find health, wholeness, and fulfillment within his or her limitations.

My goal as a healer is to help *you* find your fulfillment, too—as the person God created you to be.

So please don't misunderstand anything that I've said in this book as a blanket promise of perfect physical health. You'll know perfect health only in the resurrection. Believe me, at seventy-plus years old I'm not the same physically as I was at thirty!

If your situation is something like Eddie's, I won't even offer you pity. Through the years I've learned not to pity patients who must learn to live with serious physical limitations. Oh, I've cried with and for some of them. But I respect each individual too much to encourage a "poor me" attitude which will rob him or her of the joy of finding fulfillment.

I know that each individual truly is special. For each of us, fulfillment is found in making the most of our God-given potential.

Eddie's life was brief. He was limited by a terrible disease. But he enjoyed a fuller and more fulfilling life than many with mere physical health. When you live to the full within your limitations, as Eddie did, believe me, you are truly well.

But with this said, I want to return to the thesis of this book. It's this. *We are in much better health, and heal much more quickly, if our attitude and choices allow our God-given immune system to ward off invaders, and repair any damage illness has done.*

Meet George ━━━━━━━━━

I met George early in my medical career. He was a member of Seattle's police department. When I first met him he was driving a prowler car, and I would see him at various emergencies. We got to know each other meeting in the emergency rooms, and it seemed natural through the years that our paths kept crossing.

George was tall and big-boned, a man who absolutely radiated health, someone you'd want on your side in a fight. I became his doctor, and the doctor of his beautiful wife and daughter.

As the years passed George developed heart disease, and then acute leukemia.

His attitude was terrific. He was never too sick to be happy or to tell a good story. He was always thinking about the other person.

When he was hospitalized, his hematologist (a doctor specializing in diseases of the blood) told me his chances of recovery were slim. I spent some time with George, and we had a great talk, sharing the old times and talking about the world. In that hospital room George let me know how much our friendship had meant to him, and how much my faith was an inspiration to him. We affirmed each other and prayed together.

At that time no one knew whether or not his medication was going to do any good. But in two weeks George was much better and up and around.

I'm happy to say that last New Year's Day George phoned me, and we had a great visit. He's lost none of his dependence on God, and praises the Lord continually. He says, "It's the only way we're going to get out of this mess."

What a great attitude to have.

And what a testimony to the healing power of a healthy spirit. For a healthy spirit leads us into the very presence of God, and God is the Giver of life, the

Sustainer of life, and the Restorer of life. Right relationship with Him is the true spiritual secret of being well.

Getting Well and Staying Well ══════════

For a moment now let's review the spiritual secrets that I've shared with you in this book.

Each is based on a simple assumption. God has created wonderful internal systems designed to give us physical health. These systems work most efficiently when relieved of the excess stress that comes from unhealthy attitudes and unwise personal choices. My spiritual secrets, developed and tested through my years of medical practice, focus on helping you build the attitudes and make the choices that lead to vital good health. My secrets show you how to develop a lifestyle in which body, soul, and spirit will be in harmony, a condition that helps each of us to be well.

What then are the secrets I've shared with you?

1. *Understand and accept God as a God of love.* Fear of God, a nagging sense of guilt, the notion that God is punishing you when you are sick, are real deterrents to recovery.

The fact is that God loves you so much that He gave His only Son to die for you. Through Jesus you are a forgiven person. Yes, you will sin. And you will fall short. But God has already dealt with your sins and failures at the cross.

You can anchor yourself in the certainty that God does love you. Illness is not evidence that you have been abandoned by your Lord.

2. *Deepen your personal relationship with God by daily communication.* We each need a daily "Lone Time" with God. We need to quiet our hearts before Him, to listen to His Word, to nurture our spirits by communing with His Spirit. As you seek God, He draws close to you and brings with Him the healing gift of inner peace.

3. *Find a primary care physician whom you trust.* Feeling confident and comfortable about medical care is a vital element in recovery. As a doctor, I have learned to think of myself as God's minister of healing to the ill. We each need a relationship with a doctor we trust, who can be God's agent of healing in our lives.

4. *Develop a truly Christian hope.* Christian hope is relational. We confidently trust ourselves to God, knowing that He cares for us and plans to do us good.

Christian hope is not fixed on a particular outcome. Christian hope comes as we consciously place ourselves in God's hands, relying on His wisdom and His love to do what is best for us. As we learn to hope in God, our anxieties and fears are released and our spirits find peace.

5. *Make responsible lifestyle choices.* This means on the one hand that you will choose *not* to stress your body by abusing it with substances like tobacco, alcohol, and drugs. It also means that you will choose not to stress your spirit by abusing yourself with immoral or wicked choices. The person whose choices violate his conscience brings on an emotional and mental state that is the enemy of health and of inner peace.

6. *Make responsible diet and exercise choices.* Obesity stresses many bodily systems, and has rightly been called a "killer disease." Our bodies are temples of the Holy Spirit, and we are to treat them with respect. Good diet and exercise choices are absolute prerequisites to experiencing vital good health.

7. *Seek a spiritual renewal of your values and your priorities.* A materialistic outlook on life is closely linked with distress of the systems God has provided for maintaining health. You need to consciously choose spiritual values.

The choice of spiritual values, as these are taught in the Bible, releases us from anxieties and focuses our attention on loving relationships which bring us peace and joy. When your priorities become those God has established for His creatures, your spirit, soul, and body are in harmony, and you are free to be well.

Miracles Every Day

As a Christian I do believe in miracles. As a doctor I've seen healings which simply cannot be medically explained.

But my idea of miracles includes far more than such unexplained events.

I see *life* as a miracle. Life is a direct gift from God, and is miraculously sustained by the amazing physical systems God has provided to keep us well. For me, every recovery is a miracle. The good health that I and millions more experience is a miracle as well.

So to me, the spiritual secrets that I've shared with you seem simply a part of this wonderful miracle of life.

As you live as God intends us to live, applying the spiritual truths so in harmony with His Word, *you* will experience the miracle. And be well.

Thought and Discussion Questions

Chapter 1 ═══════

1. Think about a time in your life when you felt especially healthy and well. What was happening in your life at that time?

2. Have you ever recovered from a serious sickness to the surprise of your doctors? Have friends had this experience? How do you explain what happened?

3. What do you think Dr. Johnson means by "the power of a healthy spirit"? Is your spirit a healthy one? Why or why not?

4. What are you hoping for from your reading (and discussion of) this book?

Chapter 2 ═══════

1. Dr. Johnson begins this chapter by telling about Sharon. How has your life been *like* and *unlike* hers?

2. Do you agree or disagree: "Our state of health really depends on our genetic makeup." How does Dr. Johnson feel about this idea?

3. How are mind, body, and spirit related to the healthy functioning of that critical *immune system* which God has provided for human beings?

4. Why are miracles in a biblical sense usually unnecessary for recovery and general good health?

Chapter 3 ═══════

1. When you've been sick, have you felt that God is punishing you or has abandoned you? If Dr. Johnson

were sitting down with you in your living room, what would he say to help you with those feelings?

2. What does a sense of security in our relationship with God contribute to our recovery? How does it make a difference?

3. What five words would you choose to describe God and His attitude toward human beings? What words do you think Dr. Johnson would choose?

4. Is it all right to feel afraid and guilty sometimes? Why is the *sometimes* so important in this sentence?

5. Describe any "Lone Time" practices of your own. Which pattern suggested by Dr. Johnson would you like to try?

Chapter 4 ━━━━━

1. Do you feel comfortable with and confident in your present doctor(s)? What about him or her makes you feel this way?

2. Do you feel worried or lack confidence in your present doctor(s)? What about him or her makes you feel this way?

3. Why do you think Dr. Johnson insists that "feeling comfortable and confident about your medical care is vital for your recovery"?

4. Which ideas in this chapter about finding a good primary care physician make the most sense to you?

Chapter 5 ━━━━━

1. Dr. Johnson says that "we have a guardian against the harmful effects of stress and the destructive effects of fear." How would you describe this guardian?

2. Can you see anything on the stress chart on p. 82 that may be linked to an illness you have now or are recovering from?

3. How important do some doctors now believe is the "faith factor" in recovery from illness? How important do you believe it is?

4. Is there any basis on which you can have hope? What is that basis? What, really, is "hope"?

5. Find one Bible verse which assures that you are loved or that you can memorize as a foundation for hope.

Chapter 6 ══════════

1. If you were to take a "healthy lifestyle" quiz, how would you score? *High* (very healthy) or *low* (unhealthy)? What would account for your score?

2. Dr. Johnson does not call social drinking of alcohol a sin. But what *is* his attitude toward drinking? Why does he feel as he does?

3. Dr. Johnson includes a true story told by Dr. William Wilson of Duke University to illustrate the impact of moral choices on health. What is the problem with immorality?

4. What is the solution for persons who have already made bad choices?

Chapter 7 ══════════

1. How close are you to the *desirable weight* shown on the updated chart on p. 117?

2. What is your greatest eating problem? How did that problem develop? What have you tried to do about it in the past? How successful have you been?

3. Sit down with a friend or family member and plan *two weeks* of meals you like, working from Dr. Johnson's "Lifetime Eating" plan. How difficult would it be to use these fourteen daily diets for a period of three months as a "test" of healthy eating?

4. How hard would it be to begin vigorous family walks after supper? Or to find a partner to walk with you at another time?

Chapter 8

1. How are "spiritual renewal" and health related?

2. What evidence would others see in your life that you have experienced a spiritual renewal? What evidence that you *need* spiritual renewal?

3. Comparing characteristics of "materialistic" and "spiritual" people, fill in these blanks: "I would say that I am basically _____, because _____ ."

4. According to p. 140, what happens in the materialistic person, and how does this affect his immune system?

5. Read Matthew 6:24–34. What would it take for you to live the way Jesus recommends?